Case Studies in
Emergency Medicine

Case Studies in Emergency Medicine

Second Edition

Howard A. Freed, M.D.
Director, Residency Program, and
Associate Director,
Department of Emergency Medicine,
Albany Medical College,
Albany, New York

Frederic W. Platt, M.D.
Clinical Associate Professor of Medicine,
University of Colorado School of Medicine;
Attending Physician,
Presbyterian/St. Luke's Hospitals,
Denver, Colorado

Dan Mayer, M.D.
Associate Director for Undergraduate Education,
Department of Emergency Medicine,
Albany Medical College,
Albany, New York

Little, Brown and Company
Boston/Toronto/London

Library of Congress Catalog Card No. 90-63467

ISBN 0-316-70971-9

Printed in the United States of America

RRD-VA

Contents

Preface

Case Studies in Emergency Medicine by Frederic W. Platt first appeared in the early 1970s, years before emergency medicine was an approved medical specialty. It was a small but inspirational book and a real factor in causing at least two young physicians to choose emergency medicine as a career. Those two physicians have since grown older and become the editors of the second edition. We were able to tempt Dr. Platt into assisting us with the revision. We would like to thank Dr. Platt, a gifted teacher, for inspiring us to try to do for others what he did for us.

The only nationally recognized Core Content for medical student education in emergency medicine was drawn up by the Society of Teachers of Emergency Medicine (STEM) and published in May, 1985, in *Annals of Emergency Medicine,* about a decade after the first edition of this book appeared. Every item in that Core Content is covered in this edition (see Appendix for details).

This book is intended for medical students, nurses, paramedics, residents, and practicing physicians. It has been designed so that it can be used as an introductory text for a medical student course in emergency medicine—to be read in its entirety within a month. We stress concepts in the context of interesting cases and have not attempted to be encyclopedic.

Trying to choose a career in medicine is like trying to choose a college while in high school. It is a large step that requires a decision based, inevitably, on too little information. You never really know in detail what you are getting into until you are far past the decision point. One reason we have written this book is to try to convey to those considering emergency medicine as a career what it is like to practice our specialty. The cases are arranged not by body system, but in a random sequence similar to what one might encounter working in a busy emergency department. The cases themselves are real.

H. A. F.

D. M.

A Note on the References

Each case in this book has three types of references. The first is our favorite, basic, introductory *textbook chapter* on each subject. They are chosen from major emergency medicine textbooks. To ensure that the reader will have easy access to these references, we have limited our selections to these four commonly found books:

Tintinalli, J. E., Krome, R. L., and Ruiz, E. (eds.). *Emergency Medicine, A Comprehensive Study Guide,* 2nd edition. New York: McGraw-Hill, 1988.

Rosen, P. (ed.). *Emergency Medicine,* 2nd edition. St. Louis: Mosby, 1988.

Schwartz, G. R., et al. (eds.). *Principles and Practice of Emergency Medicine,* 2nd edition. Philadelphia: Saunders, 1986.

Fleisher, G., and Ludweig, S. (eds.). *Textbook of Pediatric Emergency Medicine,* 2nd edition. Baltimore: Williams & Wilkins, 1988.

Following the textbook reference is a more extensive, up-to-date *review article* of each subject. In those few cases where a recent review article was not available, we substituted a current *subspecialty textbook chapter.*

Last, we have included one or more *additional references* of interest.

Contributors

George L. Cooper, M.S.N., R.N., C.F.N.P.
William Fisher, M.D.
Howard A. Freed, M.D.
Charles Graffeo, M.D.
Bilal Kattan, M.D.
Peter Kelly, M.D.
Dan Mayer, M.D.
Rachel Michaud, M.S.
Frederic W. Platt, M.D.
Greer Pomeroy, M.D.
Philip Rabinowitz, M.D.
Kevin Reilly, M.D.
Richard Salluzzo, M.D.
David Salo, M.D.
Howard Snyder, M.D.
Leonard Teitz, M.D.
Shari Welch, M.D.

Case Studies in
Emergency Medicine

Notice

The indications and dosages of all drugs in this book have been recommended in the medical literature and conform to the practices of the general medical community. The medications described do not necessarily have specific approval by the Food and Drug Administration for use in the diseases and dosages for which they are recommended. The package insert for each drug should be consulted for use and dosage as approved by the FDA. Because standards for usage change, it is advisable to keep abreast of revised recommendations, particularly those concerning new drugs.

Case 1 Vital Signs Stable, Speaking Italian

We received a radio call from a local rescue squad telling us that they had picked up a male in his forties from a one-car automobile accident. His vital signs were "stable," and they had fully immobilized him to prevent head, neck, or body movement. They added that he had been unconscious and unresponsive to all stimuli, but after ten minutes he awoke and spoke in Italian. The rescue squad brought him into the emergency department with two large-bore intravenous lines that they had started running at a "wide open" rate. The damage to his car was severe.

In the trauma room, the patient's vital signs were normal. His blood pressure was 110/60, pulse 104, and respirations 20. He was alert and answered questions in English. His eyes were open and his pupils were equal and reactive to light. A strong odor of alcohol was on his breath. He complained of chest and abdominal pains. He stated that he was 48-years old and in excellent health with no medical problems. Whenever asked for details about the accident, he began speaking in an unintelligible language. When the paramedics heard this, they identified it as the speech that they had called "Italian."

His chest was tender over the sternum, but his heart and lungs were normal. Abdominal exam showed diffuse tenderness. He was awake and alert, and other than some bruises, the rest of exam was entirely normal. X-rays were obtained and all were negative.

Blood samples were sent for arterial blood gas, complete blood count, glucose, electrolytes, BUN, amylase, clotting profile, type and cross match for 6 units, alcohol level, and drug screen. He was removed from restraints after his neck and back x-rays were read as normal. Although he was quite coherent during the evaluation, questions about his accident still led to incomprehensible answers, and when queried he admitted to be speaking in tongues. With further questioning about his religious beliefs, he became angry and agitated. After fifteen minutes of lying quietly on the stretcher, he suddenly jumped up and pulled out his intravenous lines. He tore one intravenous

1

line in the middle of the tubing, and as he ran naked from the room he dripped a trail of blood. Five security guards subdued him and tied him to his bed. The staff psychiatrist was asked to see him, and he told of having driven into a tree because God had told him to kill himself.

How much training do emergency medical technicians (EMTs) have before they are allowed to infuse large amounts of intravenous fluid prior to the patient being evaluated by a physician?

Is forcible treatment of a trauma patient ever justifiable, and how should it be done?

Is there any significance to a "one-car accident"?

DISCUSSION   Most victims of automobile accidents are treated at the scene by emergency medical technicians (EMTs). Treatment usually includes splinting with a rigid cervical collar, and straps or sandbags keep them from moving their necks. They are often strapped onto a long spine board. Many emergency medical services (EMS) systems also have standing orders that if the patient is hypotensive or if the mechanism of injury suggests a high likelihood of serious internal trauma, the Military Anti-Shock Trousers (MAST) should be placed on the patient. This may be done in the field for prophylactic reasons and then only inflated if the patient's blood pressure drops below 100 mm Hg. In addition to stabilization of the spine and a rapid infusion of fluids, this patient was given high-flow oxygen by the EMT who picked him up. Basic level EMTs are trained to recognize most obvious life-threatening emergencies and to provide immediate stabilization. Advanced EMTs are trained to recognize more subtle presentations of emergencies and provide treatments such as intubation, defibrillation, initiation of intravenous therapy with fluids and drugs, and needle thoracostomy for tension pneumothorax. Basic EMT training requires about 100 hours, and advanced EMTs may spend up to 2000 hours in training.

This case was complicated by the patient's violence toward the ED staff and his irrational behavior. Generally any patient whom the staff think *might* be suicidal can be held involuntarily and physically restrained if necessary. Patients who are unable to make a rational decision about their care due to acute organic brain syndrome risk death or disability if they leave the ED. Laws on involuntary treatment vary somewhat from state to state, but all accept the principle of therapeutic restraint.

To avoid staff injury, we recommend a team of at least six members when it is necessary to restrain patients who are overtly violent. Sedative medication should be used sparingly in the multiple-trauma patient. Violent trauma patients occasionally need to be paralyzed to undergo potentially life-saving procedures such as intubation or head computed tomography (CT) scanning, but paralysis should never be used as a form of behavior control.

As a last comment, the word *stable* means unchanging or enduring. It does not mean "normal." So we may find a patient's vital signs to be quite abnormal but stable (e.g., long-standing blood pressure of 240/120), or quite normal but unstable (e.g., blood pressure of 120/70 in a patient who is beginning to hemorrhage). If we mean normal, we should say normal. Saying "stable" sometimes acts to reassure us inappropriately.

REFERENCES

Textbook   Rosen. Pp. 12–14, 1835–1844.

Review Article   Parsons, M. Fits and other causes of loss of consciousness while
                      driving. *Q. J. Med.* 1986;58(227):295–303.

Additional   Schmidt, C. W., et al. Suicide by vehicular crash. *Am. J. Psychi-*
Reference   *atry* 1977;134:175–178.

                      Stark, G., et al. Patients who initially refuse prehospital evalua-
                      tion and/or therapy. *Am. J. Emerg. Med.* 1990;8:509–511.

Case 2 Multiple Somatic Complaints

A 38-year-old woman presented to the triage nurse complaining of fatigue. She stated that this had gone on for several years on and off but had worsened over the past few days. The triage nurse correctly determined that the patient had no immediate threat to life or limb, and had her register with the clerk while assigning her an empty stretcher in a booth. Shortly after this, another nurse began to perform a nursing assessment of the patient. After this had been completed, the nurse told a junior medical resident that this patient had multiple problems and that the nurse could not quite figure out what her main problem was. Her vital signs were normal.

The resident went in, introduced himself to the patient, and obtained the following history: The patient had muscle aches and fatigue for the past ten years. She noted no specific pattern to these but thought that they frequently were related to certain foods, and she wondered about an allergy to wheat or eggs. She had intermittent chest pain, dull in nature and related neither to rest nor exertion and sometimes associated with shortness of breath. Occasionally she was short of breath without chest pain. She also had frequent headaches that were frontal in nature and relieved, usually, by acetaminophen, but she occasionally required an injection of a painkiller in the emergency department. Her vision had been changing over the past two or three years, and she had a syncopal episode a few months before but did not tell anyone about it (at the time she had no physician or health insurance). She had frequent nausea and thought it might be related also to food ingestions although not clearly wheat or eggs. She also had occasional crampy abdominal pain associated with either diarrhea or constipation but occasionally with normal bowel movements. She had urinary frequency without dysuria and complained of missing periods and of heavy periods but ascribed this to a fibroid tumor she was told about eight years prior. She noted a weight gain and loss on and off during these years, but never more than 4 or 5 pounds at a time. She admitted to having swelling of her abdomen and occasionally her feet and hands. She took many vitamins and a thyroid pill every other day and a water pill three times a week. She had been to various doctors over this period, but none of them had ever been able to help her for any period of time. She said she was sick of being sick.

The resident's examination showed no abnormalities.

The puzzled resident ordered a CBC, glucose, BUN, electrolytes, and also drew a computerized profile, thyroid function studies, and rheumatoid profile (ANA, VDRL, RA factor, ESR). The first tests came back normal, and he was about to send the patient out with a followup appointment to the medical clinic (not his own) when the nurse asked him if he thought that the patient was depressed. A brief argument ensued during which the resident told the nurse that the patient was a "crock." The attending physician on duty was asked his opinion.

He questioned the patient briefly about sleep patterns and depressive symptoms. She admitted difficulty in getting to sleep, early morning waking, and periods of crying easily. She also admitted to marital stress and job problems with her husband. She had been depressed about her illness and occasionally felt like she wanted to die by taking a bottle of pills, and admitted that she felt that way earlier in the day.

The attending reassured her that all steps would be taken to look for an organic cause of her illness, but meanwhile a pressing need was for a psychological evaluation to be performed, and the effects of the multiple symptoms on her emotional state needed to be treated. She agreed to be seen immediately by the psychiatry resident.

What is a "positive review of systems"?

How do you evaluate and treat a patient with a masked depression?

What is the role of the laboratory in the emergency department evaluation of patients with multiple somatic complaints?

DISCUSSION   Some patients will claim to have an astounding number of symptoms. Sometimes they only bring forth this array of symptoms when specifically asked. Terms we use to describe such patients are *multiple somatic complaints* and a *positive review of systems*. As physicians, we should avoid name calling. It does no good to label the patient a "crock"; it serves no useful therapeutic purpose for the patient and makes effective patient care almost impossible.

Patients with these types of complaints are obviously hard to diagnose. In a young person, these may be due to depression, overwork, failing relationships, major unresolved decisions, chronic anxiety, malingering, or the psychiatric syndrome known as somatization disorder. Some other illnesses will produce a multiplicity of symptoms. Infections such as mononucleosis or hepatitis, rheumatic or endocrine disorders, toxic exposures, and occasionally tumors may present with multiple vague symptoms, but these can usually be referred to one or a group of organ systems. In geriatric patients, vague multiple complaints can also be the presentation of cardiac, renal, or hepatic failure; drug effects; or anemia. Drug abuse, common among many young adults, may cause fatigue or other vague symptoms. The examiner must use the correct contemporary terminology to obtain an accurate history. Patients who deny drug use may admit to the use of analgesics, sedatives, tranquilizers, birth control pills, and laxatives. A patient who denies "using drugs" may admit to "doing coke or smack" (cocaine or heroin) or "popping pills."

Although true medical emergencies can exist in this setting, a more common emergency is the depressed and suicidal patient who presents with organic symptoms and may at first deny psychopathology.

To help rule out organic illness in a patient like this, it would be reasonable to obtain laboratory studies such as a chest x-ray, ECG, urinalysis, complete blood count, biochemical survey (e.g., for hepatic enzymes, calcium, potassium, bilirubin, BUN) and a sedimentation rate. If these are all negative, the patient can be reassured that there is no sign of life-threatening systemic disease.

It should also be explained to the patient that correct therapy must await correct diagnosis. Too often patients are sent home without therapy, sometimes being told that "nothing is wrong," "everything is all right," or "the illness must be in your head." This is a disservice to the patient and the medical profession. The principle that correct treatment requires correct diagnosis, and that sometimes this takes more examinations and lab studies, must be explained to patients. At the same time, the physician must be alert for signs of depression and possible suicide risk in patients who present with these symptoms as a sign of psychological illness.

The resident physician in this case was misled by the patient's rambling history and thought that he should be able to discover the diagnosis. He became frustrated when this seemed impossible. The attending physician was able to recognize the apparently aimless nature of the patient's complaints, and focused on questioning for somatic symptoms of depressive illness. The common early symptoms of depression include anxiety, insomnia (especially early morning wakening, difficulty getting to sleep, or waking frequently during the night), fatigue, change in appetite (either increase or decrease), crying spells, and an overtly depressed feeling. The patient should be asked if she had felt depressed or if she felt like killing herself or hurting herself. A common misconception is that by asking these questions, it may "give the patient an idea," and render her more likely to commit suicide. In truth, most of these people want help and just need someone to ask the right questions.

Any patient who is depressed and for whom you have any doubts about suicide risk should be referred to a psychiatrist for an immediate evaluation. We tell our patients that this is a rule in our department and does not mean that they are crazy (a common misconception), but only that we feel there is a psychological component to their illness. It helps to emphasize to the patient that the psychiatric evaluation does not mean a diagnosis of mental illness is being made, but it serves as an entry into a counseling setting.

REFERENCES

Textbook   Rosen. Pp. 32–33, 226, 1872–1874.

Review Article   Gerson, S., and Bassuk, E. Psychiatric emergencies: An overview. *Am. J. Psychiatry* 1980;137:1–11.

Additional   Monson, R. A., and Smith G. R., Jr. Somatization disorder in
Reference   primary care. *N. Engl. J. Med.* 1983;308:1464–1465.

Case **3** Sprain?

A 30-year-old male school teacher arrived in the emergency department complaining of having sprained his left wrist while playing tennis two days earlier. He was rather proud of his tennis game and stated that he had been reaching for a "winner" when he fell forcibly onto the outstretched palm of his hand. He had moderate swelling and there was pain with any movement of the wrist joint. The pain was most severe when he attempted to write anything on the blackboard.

The patient was a pleasant young man with physical findings limited to his wrist. On inspection, the left wrist showed diffuse swelling in comparison to the contours of the normal right side. The wrist felt spongy and full distal to the end of the radius. The patient localized the area of maximum tenderness to a point distal to the radial styloid in the location of the "anatomic snuffbox." He had a great deal of pain when he tried to pronate or supinate his hand against resistance.

What is a sprain? A strain?

How should this patient be managed?

DISCUSSION   A *sprain* is defined as an injury to one or more ligaments supporting a joint in which the joint retains its anatomic alignment.
The sprain can be classified as first degree (mild ligamentous
damage, moderate pain and swelling); second degree (moderate ligamentous damage, marked pain and swelling, but stable
joint); or third degree (severe ligament damage, and unstable
joint). The degree of swelling and pain around an injured joint
has a strong correlation with the amount of ligamentous damage.

The diagnosis of a joint sprain is really one of exclusion. It is
diagnosed when all bony injuries in and around a specified joint
have been excluded. When the location of maximum pain and
swelling is over a known ligament, and a fracture has been
ruled out, then a sprain can be diagnosed. Third-degree sprains
are differentiated from second-degree sprains with stress x-ray
views of a joint. These views are usually too painful to perform
in routine emergency department management and are usually
delayed until the swelling has subsided three to four days later.

Most first-degree sprains have a benign course, but a missed
third- or severe second-degree sprain can cause years of pain
and disability. Operative management is sometimes necessary
in these cases. All patients with sprains should be referred to a
primary care physician or orthopedist for followup.

The term *strain* describes overexercise or overstretch of a
muscle or group of muscles resulting in pain and short-term
disability. For example, the common presentation of back
"strain" is usually a complex condition involving multiple muscles that support the spine. It can be precipitated by a single
episode of heavy lifting lasting only seconds, by isometric con-
traction such as a "whiplash" injury, or by normal activity.

This case illustrates the necessity of performing a careful
physical exam with a working knowledge of the underlying
anatomy. The patient had maximum tenderness over the navicular (scaphoid) bone. A fracture in this bone is sometimes
impossible to see on the standard x-ray views of the wrist, and a
special "navicular view" should be requested. Nonetheless,
even with the navicular view, fractures may only be detected
seven to ten days later when persistent wrist pain leads to a
followup x-ray, and bone resorption in the fracture site makes it
visible on x-ray. Any patient with point tenderness over the
navicular should be treated as a navicular fracture until followup evaluation rules it out.

In this case, the navicular view was requested in addition to
the standard views, and a transverse fracture through the waist
of the navicular bone was clearly seen. The patient was immo-

bilized in a thumb spica cast for six weeks and had good union of the fracture site with no development of the painful aseptic necrosis that can follow fractures of this bone.

Other common injuries masquerade as sprains of other joints. A neck or back "sprain" may be a vertebral compression fracture, metastatic disease in the spine, meningitis, or even a subarachnoid hemorrhage. A shoulder "sprain" may be an acromioclavicular separation, a rotator cuff tear, a humeral or sternoclavicular dislocation, or even a myocardial infarction. A knee "sprain" may be a medial or lateral meniscus tear, a septic joint, a Baker's cyst, a tibial plateau fracture, gout, or may be referred pain from some disease in the hip.

So, the moral of this story is be suspicious, take a careful history, and think and examine anatomically any patient who complains of a "sprained" anything.

REFERENCES

Textbook Tintinalli. Pp. 882–892.

Review Article Green, D. F. The "sprained wrist." *Am. Fam. Prac.* 1979; 19(4):114–122.

Additional References Simon, R. R., and Koenigsknecht, S. J. The Carpals. In *Orthopedics In Emergency Medicine, The Extremities*. New York, Appleton-Century-Crofts, 1982. Pp 74–89.

Dobyns, J., and Linscheid, R. L. Fractures and Dislocations of the Wrist. In C. A. Rockwood and P. Green (eds.), *Fractures In Adults,* volume 1. Philadelphia, Lippincott, 1984. Pp. 411–420, 450–509.

Harris, T. H., and Harris, W. H. Hand and Wrist. In *The Radiology of Emergency Medicine*, 2nd edition. Baltimore, Williams & Wilkins, 1981. Pp. 250–292.

Case 4 Refusing Treatment

Paramedics were called to the home of a 69-year-old woman. Her daughter had noticed a change in her mother's behavior over the past several days and tried to get her to the doctor. The day before, the daughter had called the ambulance twice and they left both times after the mother refused transport to the hospital.

The paramedics attempted to get vital signs, but the patient refused, therefore, the only one they were able to obtain was a respiratory rate of 24 per minute. The patient was agitated and appeared upset at the presence of the paramedics in her home. She was answering their questions appropriately and still refusing to go to the hospital even for a "check up." The medics contacted their hospital base station for medical control.

The medical control physician agreed with the medics' assessment that the patient should be seen in the hospital. He was unsure of the degree of impairment of the patient's ability to decide for herself whether or not she needed treatment. He asked to speak to the woman's daughter and ascertained that the patient's behavior was truly unusual and that the change had been abrupt, over only a few days. He then ordered the paramedics to bring the patient to the hospital against her will, stating "You're a lot bigger than she is."

In the ambulance they placed an oxygen mask on the patient. Shortly after, she stated that she felt better and that she was glad they were taking her to the hospital. Evaluation in the emergency department disclosed a bilateral pneumonia and hypoxemia. She made an uneventful recovery.

Do all patients have a right to refuse treatment?

When can patients be held against their will for treatment?

What constitutes assault in the medical setting?

DISCUSSION   This patient presented with an acute organic brain syndrome
                   secondary to hypoxia. This diagnosis was made by her daugh-
                   ter who noted that her behavior was different from usual. In
                   older patients, this may be the only clue to an acute underlying
                   medical problem and should never be passed off as being de-
                   mentia until all treatable causes of acute mental status changes
                   have been ruled out.

                   In this case, the first two ambulances allowed this woman to
                   sign herself out from medical care against medical advice
                   (AMA). In the prehospital setting, this is commonly referred to
                   as *refusal of medical attention (RMA)*. Allowing patients who
                   have requested medical care to sign out without receiving an
                   evaluation by a physician is a potentially dangerous practice.
                   The legal liability for abandonment is great, especially if it can
                   be proven that the patient may not have understood the ram-
                   ifications of refusing care.

                   Patients, in general, have the right to refuse any medical care
                   offered. In order to refuse medical help, the patient must be
                   "competent" to make this decision. Competency, or the lack of
                   it, can only be determined by a judge. An operational medical
                   definition requires that the patient fully understand the ramifica-
                   tions of her decision to refuse care. Most patients can be given
                   the facts, asked questions to determine their understanding of
                   the facts, and then sign a statement attesting to this understand-
                   ing. The documentation of these cases is extremely important,
                   and the signing of the AMA statement should be witnessed by
                   at least one other staff person and, if possible, a member of the
                   patient's family.

                   Some patients cannot be assumed to understand all the ram-
                   ifications of their refusals. These include any patient who is
                   intoxicated or who has hypoxia, acidosis, or another metabolic
                   derangement. These patients should be held for treatment
                   against their will. Of course the problem at the scene is knowing
                   which patient has one of these problems. We can seldom be
                   sure. An abnormal vital sign might alert us to the presence of a
                   worrisome metabolic or cardiovascular-pulmonary derange-
                   ment, but what angry person, resisting unwarranted intrusion,
                   will not have a tachycardia or elevated blood pressure?

                   Patients who are suicidal or homicidal may also be held
                   against their will until a psychiatrist says that they no longer
                   represent a threat to themselves or others. Physical restraint
                   may be needed in these cases.

                   A patient can bring suit against a physician for treatment
                   rendered against the patient's wishes. The complaint is a civil

charge of assault, and the plaintiff must prove that the physician acted with wanton disregard for the patient's safety or in a malicious manner. The patient must also prove that damages resulted from this treatment. Usually the damages that result from proper restraint of a patient are less than damages resulting from not treating the patient. Additionally, lack of treatment can result in a poor outcome and lead to a suit for medical malpractice. This has occurred in cases of intoxicated patients being allowed to leave the emergency department AMA without adequate diagnosis (e.g., subdural hematomas, cervical spine fractures) who then have progression of their illness or injury resulting in impairment or death.

REFERENCES
Textbook

Rosen. Pp. 31–34.

Review Article

Dunn, J. D. Risk management in emergency medicine. *Emerg. Med. Clin. North Am.* 1987;5:51–69.

Additional References

Fastow, J. Medical malpractice and emergency medicine: The crisis of the 1980's (editorial). *Am. J. Emerg. Med.* 1985;6:571–573.

Holroyd, B., et al. Pre-hospital patients refusing care. *Ann. Emerg. Med.* 1988;17:957–963.

Lipowski, Z. J. Delerium in the elderly patient. *N. Engl. J. Med.* 1989;320:578–582.

Appelbaum, B. S., and Roth, L. H. Patients who refuse treatment in medical hospitals. *J.A.M.A.* 1983;250:1296–1301.

Case 5 Terrible Sore Throat

A 26-year-old woman came to the emergency department at 7 P.M. with the following story: She had been ill for four days, suffering with a "terribly sore throat," fatigue, and fever. She felt "all in." There was no significant past history, and she had been well until four days before. The emergency physician examined her and noted large tonsils covered by purulent exudate. She had a fever of 101°F and the doctor thought that she might have slight splenomegaly. The upper cervical lymph nodes were large and tender, but she did not have significant lymphadenopathy elsewhere. The doctor said that he thought she had a streptococcal throat infection, but that mononucleosis was also a real possibility. He cultured her throat, obtained a Monospot test, and prescribed ampicillin four times a day for ten days.

Two days later she returned again to the ED and said that she felt still worse. Her fever had not subsided, the throat was only marginally better, and worst of all, she thought that her entire body was swelling up. The physician checked her throat culture from two days before and told her that she did indeed have strep, that she would surely feel better in a day or two, and encouraged her to continue with the ampicillin. He told her that nothing was wrong with her skin and that the sensation of "swelling up" was probably nothing to worry about.

Three days later she made an emergency appointment to see a physician in the community. She said that she thought she was dying and that she was worse and worse each day. The fever had risen to 104°F, she was very weak, and her skin was bright red. On examination the most remarkable finding was indeed her skin. It was markedly edematous, red, and hot all over her body. She was 20 pounds over her usual weight, and the doctor surmised that it was all fluid. She appeared very toxic and was, in addition, very angry about what she considered to be cavalier treatment by the ED doctor who had "refused to hear her complaint of swelling" on the previous visit. The physician called the hospital laboratory and found that indeed the throat culture had been positive for group A, beta-hemolytic streptococci but that the Monospot test was also positive. He stopped her ampicillin, placed her on high-dose corticosteroids, and she made an uneventful recovery over the next week.

What is the relationship between mononucleosis and ampicillin?

What should your strategy be when your patient is very concerned about a physical finding or a symptom that you cannot see on your exam? Or when you and the patient disagree about the diagnosis or the treatment?

DISCUSSION Patients with mononucleosis frequently develop rashes when treated with ampicillin or one of its derivatives. Some authors show as many as 95% of such patients develop erythema, pruritus, or a maculopapular rash when exposed to ampicillin. The drug has even been suggested, perhaps facetiously, as a diagnostic test for the disease. Since ampicillin is no more useful for streptococcal tonsillitis than penicillin and has this unfortunate complication in patients with mononucleosis, and since other bacterial infections of the tonsils (e.g., *Haemophilus influenzae*) are rare in adults, it should probably not be one of your favorite drugs for bacterial pharyngitis or tonsillitis. A newer derivative, amoxicillin and clavulinic acid, interferes with the bacterial beta lactamases that inactivate penicillin. This combination drug may have a role that ampicillin itself lacks, but we would still not recommend it for this patient.

This patient was convinced that her ED physician had refused to hear her complaint. She thought that he treated her concern with disdain and that his arrogance led him to continue her antibiotic several days further, causing more suffering. She was mad enough to sue. When patients report that their doctor did not listen to them, they are very often right: He or she has not listened. There is no excuse for such behavior, and neither patients nor our profession has to condone it. Another possibility represents a situation that even careful, considerate physicians find themselves in frequently. The patient may tell you of a physical finding that you cannot find when you examine her. Then there is no satisfactory solution but to describe the trouble back to the patient. "We have a real dilemma here. You notice that your skin seems swollen, but I cannot identify it on my examination. You are probably sensing something that I can't pick up yet. I don't know what it means and may not be able to help until it gets even worse, so that even I can see it." It may help to tell the patient that such situations are common, that they usually solve themselves by going away before the doctor can make a diagnosis, and that sometimes they get worse and then we can figure them out. This is not really very different from the bind you find yourself in when your diagnosis or planned therapy differs from what the patient thought or expected. You have to say, "I know you thought that it would probably be wise to have a shot of penicillin for your cold. I think you are right about the diagnosis, but, unfortunately, this kind of infection doesn't respond to that sort of therapy." A discussion like this leaves the patient with the feeling that her opinion has been considered, that she has been heard, and that even if she was right, it is reasonable to go with your opinion since you are the professional in the matter.

REFERENCES

Textbook   Rosen. Pp. 1072–1082.

Review Article   Heffelfinger, D. C. Gianotti-Croti syndrome in association with Epstein-Barr virus altered by ampicillin. *Ala. Med.* 1985;27: 16–18.

Additional   Pullen, H., et al. Hypersensitivity reactions to antibacterial
References   drugs in infectious mononucleosis. *Lancet* 1967;II:1176–1178.

                          Pullen, H., et al. Hypersensitivity to the penicillins. *Lancet* 1968;II:1090.

Case 6 Seventy-Nine Years Old and Confused

A 79-year-old man with a previous diagnosis of organic brain syndrome was brought in by his relatives. They said that they had picked him up from his nursing home that morning to go to their annual summer picnic. He seemed fine except for his usual problem with memory. After lunch, he went to sit in the car to watch the softball game. Several hours later his relatives found him locked in the car, quite agitated and confused.

On physical examination, he was combative and irritable and had red, hot, dry skin. His rectal temperature was 42°C (107.6°F), pulse 160 and quite irregular, respiratory rate 24, and blood pressure 110/80. His neurologic exam showed no focal abnormality. His neck was supple. His venous pressure seemed slightly increased and he had bibasilar rales. A few petechiae were evident on his skin and, when a Foley catheter was placed, it was noted that he had very little urine output.

What is wrong with this man?

What are the common risk factors for this disorder?

What are its major complications?

What are the most important therapeutic tasks?

DISCUSSION   *Heat stroke* is defined as hyperpyrexia (temperature above 105°F) with altered mental status. It is a true medical emergency and is often seen among the elderly, the very young, those who are mentally impaired, and those with defective sweating mechanisms. Sweating may be impaired in the congenital absence of sweat glands, cystic fibrosis, and brainstem or spinal cord injuries. Certain drugs have been associated with heat stroke including anticholinergics, phenothiazines, antihistamines, tricyclic antidepressants, and amphetamines.

Complications can involve the cardiovascular system. Heart failure and pulmonary edema may be secondary to the marked increase in cardiac output in this syndrome. The patient may suffer centrilobular necrosis of the liver or acute tubular necrosis of the kidneys. There may also be rhabdomyolysis and myoglobinuria leading to renal failure, especially if the heat stroke is exercise induced (as may be seen in young athletes). Pulmonary aspiration, seizures, and coma may occur.

Laboratory abnormalities in heat stroke may include thrombocytopenia and decreased clotting factors secondary to disseminated intravascular coagulation. One may find hypoglycemia, respiratory alkalosis, or metabolic acidosis. Hyperkalemia from cell breakdown and release of potassium stores is to be anticipated.

The treatment of heat stroke requires removing the patient from the hot environment, removing clothing, and allowing evaporative cooling by applying cool or cold water to the skin surface. Unlike *hypo*thermia, where rapid external warming can be detrimental, in *hyper*thermia, aggressive external cooling is exactly what is needed. Hypoglycemia is common in this syndrome, and dextrose should be given. Since many of these patients are alcoholic, thiamine is an appropriate accompaniment. Adequate hydration and alkalinization of the urine to protect against myoglobinuric renal failure are also important. Careful attention to the hydration state is essential. Most patients with heat stroke are volume depleted, but caution must be taken to avoid fluid overload. A central venous pressure monitor may be useful. Liver function and clotting studies should be followed.

REFERENCES

Textbook Rosen. Pp. 693–715.

Review Article Shibolet, S., Lancester, M. C., and Danon, Y. Heat stroke: A review. *Aviat. Space Environ. Med.* 1976;47:280–301.

Additional Reference Knochel, J. P. Environmental heat illness: An eclectic review. *Arch. Intern. Med.* 1974;137:841–864.

Case 7 Eye Pain

A 25-year-old man came to the emergency department complaining of pain in his right eye for two weeks. He had noted copious tearing, a decrease in visual acuity, and photophobia.

He was sitting on the stretcher holding his right eye and rocking back and forth when the doctor first saw him. His visual acuity by Snellen's chart was 20/50 in the right eye (OD), 20/30 in the left eye (OS), and 20/30 when both eyes were open. His lids and lashes were normal, and no foreign body was noted when the lids were everted. There was copious tear production in the right eye. The conjunctiva of his right eye was injected, particularly near the pupil. On slit lamp examination, cells were noted in the anterior chamber. The pupil of the right eye was 2 mm in diameter and the left was 4 mm in diameter. Both were round and reactive to light. The fundi were normal.

What is the differential diagnosis for the red eye?

What "red flags" in the history and physical exam point toward a diagnosis requiring emergency ophthalmologic consultation?

DISCUSSION   The vast majority of red eyes are due to benign conditions. The differential diagnosis for a red eye includes conjunctivitis, corneal injury, anterior uveitis, scleritis, occlusion of the lacrimal system, and acute-angle closure glaucoma. Findings that suggest a malignant process are visual loss, photophobia, severe pain, abnormal pupils, and cells found in the anterior chamber.

The patient presenting with a red eye without change in visual acuity, pupillary abnormality, or problems with the anterior chamber probably has conjunctivitis. Bacterial, viral, and allergic etiologies are the most common forms. Typically, bacterial conjunctivitis produces large amounts of discharge. A gram stain of the discharge may indicate the etiology and should be done routinely in patients with copious purulent drainage. Differentiation between bacterial and viral etiologies is difficult. Because of this, most conjunctivitis patients are treated with a topical antibiotic such as 10% sodium sulfacetamide, gentamicin, or erythromycin. Several types of conjunctivitis need special mention. Neonatal conjunctivitis may be gonococcal or chlamydial, but because gonococcal conjunctivitis can lead to blindness, the infection must be considered gonococcal until proven otherwise. Treatment of gonococcal conjunctivitis should always be undertaken in the hospital with systemic antibiotics, in addition to frequent irrigation to remove purulent discharge. Vesicular lesions of the periorbital area suggest infection by herpes simplex or by varicella-zoster viruses. With herpes, the characteristic finding is the typical herpetic dendrite of the cornea seen on fluorescein exam. With either herpes simplex or varicella-zoster involvement, ophthalmologic consultation is mandated.

Corneal abrasions or ulcers are the second most common cause of "pinkeye." Visual acuity may be affected if the lesion is in the central portion of the cornea. The pupils and anterior chamber should be normal. The characteristic finding is a focal uptake of fluorescein in the area of corneal injury. A corneal foreign body is a common associated finding. Corneal injury may be caused by ultraviolet light from welding arcs, suntanning lamps, and sunlight, resulting in multiple punctate lesions over the cornea. This causes a "starry night" appearance of the cornea on fluorescein staining. Another characteristic pattern of staining is found when foreign bodies become lodged under the eyelids, producing multiple, vertically oriented corneal abrasions. Eversion of the lids to locate a foreign body is key when this pattern is identified and should be routine in your examination of painful or inflamed eyes. Treatment consists of removal of the foreign body, antimicrobial ointment, and an occlusive patch. The patch may be removed after twenty-four hours and the eye reexamined for healing, which is generally complete. If the eye is not dramatically improved by then, the patch should be replaced and the patient seen by an ophthalmologist. Of course a contact lens should not be worn on an inflamed eye, whatever the cause, until healing is complete.

Allergic conjunctivitis is often misdiagnosed as viral conjunctivitis. It should be suspected when itching and a watery discharge are prominent features and there is seasonal recurrence. Treatment should include cold compresses and topical vasoconstrictor-antihistamine eyedrops (e.g., Naphcon-A). Often the allergen is related to contact lenses, makeup, or other facial hygienic products. Discontinuation of these materials will bring about resolution of symptoms.

Anterior uveitis is a common condition resulting in a red eye and was the cause of this patient's problems. It is caused by inflammation of the iris and ciliary body producing photophobia, slight change in visual acuity, and deep, aching pain. Iritis (uveitis) should be suspected any time a red eye is treated as conjunctivitis but fails to improve promptly with treatment. On physical exam, the pupil is minimally and painfully reactive, and a ciliary blush (conjunctival injection concentrated around the pupil) may be present. Inflammatory cells floating in the anterior chamber may be seen on slit lamp exam. Treatment is aimed at dilation of the pupil to prevent formation of synechiae (adhesions of the iris to the lens). Our patient was seen later that day by an ophthalmologist who treated him with topical steroids and homatropine. Evaluation by an ophthalmologist is necessary to follow the clinical course. If there are other suggestive symptoms or a prior history of anterior uveitis, a workup for connective tissue disease is warranted.

Acute-angle closure glaucoma is an infrequent, vision-threatening entity that presents as a red eye. The patient will complain of severe pain in the affected eye. The pain may be precipitated by entering a dark room when the pupil dilates. Physical findings of note are a ciliary blush, a cloudy, poorly reactive, midposition pupil, and markedly increased intraocular pressures. Immediate therapy with 2% pilocarpine drops every fifteen minutes to constrict the pupil buys enough time to obtain emergency ophthalmologic consultation.

REFERENCES

Textbook   Schwartz. Pp. 1161–1163.

Review Article   Stock, E. L. External eye diseases. *Postgrad. Med.*
                        1985;78:102–111.

Additional   Siegel, J. D. Eye infections encountered by the pediatrician.
References   *Pediatr. Infect. Dis.* 1986;5:741–748.

                        Gittinger, J. W. Ocular Infections. In J. B. Wyngaarden and
                        L. H. Smith (eds)., *Cecil Textbook of Medicine* 18th edition.
                        Philadelphia, Saunders, 1988. P. 2294.

Case 8 "Sick All Over"

A 26-year-old woman came to the emergency department complaining of feeling "sick all over" and suddenly fainted in the triage area. She woke shortly after and was able to give the following history: She had been vomiting for several days and could not even keep water down. She also complained of a vague, diffuse abdominal pain.

On examination she was seen to be a very distressed woman who appeared to be breathing deeply but denied dyspnea. Her eyes were sunken, her skin turgor decreased, and her mucous membranes were parched.

Her temperature was 99°F, pulse 120, blood pressure 100/50, respiratory rate 36, and her neck veins were flat, suggesting a very low central venous pressure. When asked to stand up, she became faint and pale. Her abdomen was soft and had normal bowel sounds. She had no abdominal or costovertebral angle tenderness, and the rest of her examination was normal.

What do you think about asking a patient who has just fainted to stand up?

What feature of this patient requires urgent therapy at this point without any further diagnostic testing?

What might be the underlying problem?

What diagnostic tests, some easy and available at the bedside, would you do?

DISCUSSION   This patient has a low arterial blood pressure, and it will fall still lower when she sits or stands. Before standing her up, we should obtain a careful pulse and blood pressure in the supine position and then try it again in the seated position. If she has a significant fall in the mean arterial pressure when she sits up, there is no need to ask more of her.

Although it looks like a simple case of severe gastroenteritis, the patient actually has a rather classic picture of *new* diabetic ketoacidosis (DKA) with hypovolemia and dehydration. Abdominal pain, nausea, and vomiting are commonly seen in DKA. Her tachypnea is caused by her hypotension and her metabolic acidosis. Patients whose tachypnea is driven by metabolic acidosis may not sense shortness of breath. The feature of the disorder that demands urgent therapy is her hypovolemia. Eventually you will want to treat her with insulin, and perhaps with sodium bicarbonate, but right now she requires copious volumes of intravenous saline.

Two bedside tests that could help confirm your diagnosis are Chemstrips (or Dextrostix) that give a rapid gross estimate of blood sugar and a urine dipstick that will show sugar and ketones. Once you are giving the patient fluid, you will ask for more precise chemistry data including electrolytes and an arterial blood gas determination. DKA patients usually present with hyperkalemia secondary to their acidosis. Once therapy has begun, they may quickly become hypokalemic as the acidosis corrects and insulin drives sugar and potassium into cells.

We need to search for the trigger event that put our patient into ketoacidosis. A focus of infection, inappropriate cessation of insulin therapy, trauma, a myocardial infarction, and maybe even emotional stress may trigger DKA. It is reasonable to obtain a complete blood count and urinalysis, blood cultures, chest x-rays, and an ECG. Unfortunately, in many cases, we are unable to find the triggering event. Perhaps it is too subtle for us.

Normal saline is the fluid of choice and may be run in rapidly through a large-bore intravenous line. An initial hydration rate of 1000 ml over one-half hour is reasonable in a young adult. Once the potassium level begins to decline and is down into the normal range, potassium should be added to the intravenous fluid.

Insulin is usually given as a regular insulin drip at a rate of 6 to 10 units per hour after an initial bolus of 6 to 10 units. Patients with obvious infection require more insulin than those without such a disorder. When the blood sugar has decreased to about 250 mg per dl, glucose can be added to the infusion to prevent overshoot hypoglycemia. The insulin should be continued to clear circulating ketones.

REFERENCES

Textbook   Schwartz. Pp. 1069–1081.

Review Articles   Forster, D. W., and Mcgary, J. D. The metabolic derangements and treatment of diabetic ketoacidosis. *N. Engl. J. Med.* 1983; 309:159–169.

Kitabchi, A. E., and Murphy, M. B. Diabetic ketoacidosis and hyperosmolar hyperglycemic non-ketotic coma. *Med. Clin. North Am.* 1988;72:1545–1563.

Additional   Crane, E. J. Diabetic ketoacidosis: Biochemistry, physiology,
Reference   treatment and prevention. *Pediatr. Clin. North Am.* 1987;34: 935–960.

Case 9 Sexual Assault

A 35-year-old woman was brought to the emergency department by two police officers at 2 A.M. for evaluation and treatment following a sexual assault. She stated that at about 11 P.M. she was abducted by two men who beat her with their fists and forced her to have oral and vaginal intercourse. She was not sure whether ejaculation occurred. Her complaints were of abdominal, perineal, and head pain. Her last voluntary sexual intercourse was three days previously.

On examination, the patient appeared preoccupied. Her hair was in disarray and her clothes spotted with mud. She had areas of abrasion and ecchymosis about the right eye. Oral examination was unremarkable, but samples were obtained for culture (gonorrhea and chlamydia), acid phosphatase determination, and microscopic exam. She had scattered bruising over the forearms and abrasions over both knees. Her abdomen was soft with a mild, generalized tenderness. On pelvic exam, the external genitalia were normal, except for two small superficial posterior fourchette lacerations. The vaginal vault had scant amounts of white discharge that were sampled for acid phosphatase and wet mount. The bimanual exam showed mild discomfort with palpation of the uterus and adnexal structures, but no other abnormalities were found. On microscopic exam, the sample from the oral pharynx was negative, and the vaginal swab showed motile sperm.

What special steps need to be taken for legal documentation and evidence collection?

How should the problems of pregnancy and venereal disease prophylaxis be addressed?

What type of followup care should be arranged?

DISCUSSION   Care of the sexual assault victim in the ED should involve a team approach. The team should consist of the physician, a nurse, a social worker, a police officer (preferably specifically trained in rape intervention), and when needed, a psychiatrist. The primary goal of this team should be care of the patient's medical and psychiatric needs. Secondary goals of evidence collection, documentation, and reporting the alleged assault to authorities should not take precedence over the patient's care.

The history should be as complete as possible without adding to the trauma of the incident by overemphasizing the details of the assault. Preferably the history should be obtained by a single member of the team and not be repeated by other members. The date and time of both the assault and exam should appear on the chart. A brief description of the assault including the use of force, drugs, or foreign bodies, and specifics of sexual contact (oral, vaginal, or anal penetration) need to be documented. Details of personal hygiene (urination, defecation, douching, and bathing) and any clothing change since the assault need documentation. Past gynecologic history (pregnancy, last menstrual period, intercourse) and medical history should be included.

The physical examination should be thorough and should document all injuries. The clothing worn during the assault should be placed in a paper bag by the patient. The mental status of the patient at the time should be noted, including whether she is mentally competent to consent to intercourse. Pelvic exam should be documented in detail including external genitalia, appearance of the hymen (or remnant), vaginal vault, and presence of any discharge. Use of the Wood's lamp may facilitate location of dried semen, which will fluoresce.

Samples that should be gathered during the examination include:

1. Saliva from the patient on a small cotton cloth (to determine if the blood group antigens are secreted).
2. Blood sample for VDRL, beta–human chorionic gonadotropin (HCG), and type/RH.
3. Swabs from any orifice entered for acid phosphatase and a separate swab for a wet prep to be examined by the physician for sperm (motility should be documented).
4. Combings of the patient's hair and pubic hair for foreign material.
5. 10 pulled and 15 closely cropped hairs from the pubic region and a similar number from the head.

6. Gonorrhea and chlamydia cultures.
7. Fingernail scrapings.

Each of these specimens must be labeled with the patient's name, date obtained, source of the sample, and the initials of the person obtaining the sample. All samples should be placed in a sealed envelope and the chain of evidence documented on the envelope (date/time the evidence was obtained/transferred and your name/title).

Venereal disease prophylaxis should be offered to all patients who present with a history of sexual assault. Because between 40 to 90% of patients do not return for followup, venereal disease prophylaxis while the patient is in the ED is usually preferable to awaiting culture result with treatment at a later date. Prophylaxis for gonorrhea, chlamydia, and syphilis should be initiated with standard therapy. This includes 3.5 gm of oral ampicillin and 2 gm of probenecid orally and a seven-day course of doxycycline (in nonpregnant patients). In areas where penicillin-resistant gonorrhea is common, 250 mg of ceftriaxone (intramuscularly) should be given in lieu of oral ampicillin.

Counseling about human immunodeficiency virus (HIV) disease is always part of our rape treatment program. Depending on the nature of the assault, HIV blood testing may be recommended at three and six months after the encounter. Animal studies suggest that if the patient is seen within 24 hours of the assault, 6 weeks of treatment with AZT may be effective prophylaxis against the development of HIV infection in the victim.

Pregnancy prophylaxis should be discussed with all patients. All forms of prophylaxis available at this time have a relatively high incidence of side effects. Treatment options include (1) institute no therapy and wait for next menses, (2) repeat serum HCG determination in seven days and if positive consider therapeutic abortion, and (3) high-dose estrogen therapy such as two Ovral tablets bid every twelve hours for two doses plus an antiemetic such as Compazine for nausea. All "morning after" forms of therapy are effective within seventy-two hours of intercourse but are teratogenic to existing pregnancies; therefore, it is imperative that pregnancy be ruled out before initiation of therapy.

All patients should be offered intervention through an established rape crisis center.

Followup examination should be scheduled at one and six weeks, at which time repeat gonorrhea culture, syphilis serology, and pregnancy testing should be done. Psychiatric interventions and referral to a rape crisis center should be repeated as necessary at that time.

Sexual assault is a frightening experience that will change forever that person's life. The expedient delivery of health care and the humanistic treatment of the patient at the time of presentation to the ED are important first steps in restoring order to a life in disarray.

REFERENCES
Textbook   Tintinalli. Pp. 383–387.

Review Article   Kobernick, M. E., Seifert, S., and Saunders, A. B. Emergency department management of the sexual assault victim. *J. Emerg. Med.* 1985;2:205–214.

Additional   Elam, A. L., and Ray, V. G. Sexually related trauma: A review.
References   *Ann. Emerg. Med.* 1986;15:576–584.

                        Tintinalli, J. E., and Holzer, M. Clinical findings and legal resolution in sexual assault. *Ann. Emerg. Med.* 1985;14:447–453.

Case 10 Five Sick Siblings

On one hot summer afternoon, five of the seven children in one family visited a physician. They complained of abdominal pains of two days' duration. One child also had fever and diarrhea. The physician diagnosed viral gastroenteritis and suggested fluids and rest. There was no improvement during the next day, and by the following morning three of the children did not respond to voice, and the others were obviously ill. Later that day, all seven children were brought to a hospital emergency department. Two were in respiratory arrest, and the other five had various degrees of lethargy, increased respiratory secretions, increased salivation, and pupillary constriction. Two of the children died. The next day the laboratory reported that all the children had depressed serum and erythrocyte cholinesterase levels.

What sort of poisoning should have been suspected?

How is it best treated?

DISCUSSION   The presentation of a cluster of cases of a similar illness should
lead one to suspect an environmental toxic cause. Although it is
common for all the children in a household to develop a viral
gastroenteritis, it is unusual for them to all develop the symptoms at one time. Food poisoning by staphylococcal toxin is the
most common of the so-called common source illnesses that
present this way. The common thread will be that all affected
members ate the same food. Botulism will also present this way,
with the complaints related to muscular weakness, usually beginning with the ocular muscles. Carbon monoxide poisoning,
another common source illness, may initially present with abdominal pain and headache before progressing to neurologic
changes, coma, and death.

Serum and erythrocyte cholinesterase levels are depressed in
acute organophosphate poisoning, but the results of that test
may not be back soon enough to make the diagnosis. Additionally, the range of normal is so great that a level may actually
be significantly depressed from that patient's baseline and be
read as "normal." Treatment with a test dose of atropine may
make the diagnosis.

Cholinergic poisoning is characterized by the SLUDGE (Salivation, Lacrimation, Urinary incontinence, Diarrhea, Gastrointestinal irritability, and Emesis) syndrome. There can be rhonchi
and wheezes on the lung exam, the bowel sounds will be hyperactive, and bradycardia and profuse diaphoresis may be present. The most common cause of this syndrome is poisoning
with an insecticide of the organophosphate class. These agents
bind to and inactivate acetylcholinesterase, causing a symptomatic buildup of acetylcholine and a rush of cholinergic discharge. The immediate treatment is with intravenous atropine
titrated until signs of atropinization appear (the wheezing stops,
the pupils dilate, and the heart rate increases). Huge doses of
atropine, often 20 to 30 mg per hour, may be needed to control
the symptoms. In severe anticholinergic poisoning, this is followed by pralidoxime (2-PAM), a drug that removes the organophosphate from the enzyme and allows acetylcholine to be
degraded normally.

The source of the organophosphates in this case was never
definitely identified. There was some dust on equipment used
for spraying that the children were playing with. The adults,
who had not touched the equipment, were unaffected. Organophosphates are rapidly absorbed through the skin, and they
must be fully removed as quickly as possible to reduce the

amount absorbed. The powder on the skin of a victim can also pose a hazard to the rescuer.

REFERENCES

Textbook   Tintinalli. Pp. 737–741.

Review Article Mortensen, M. L. Management of acute childhood poisoning caused by selected insecticides and herbicides. *Pediatr. Clin. North Am.* 1986;33:421–445.

Additional   Midtling, J. E., et al. Clinical management of field worker
Reference   organophosphate poisoning. *West. J. Med.* 1985;142:514–518.

Case 11 Keyhole Medicine

A nurse hands you the phone and says that some woman is calling about her husband; could you please see what you can do with her. You introduce yourself and the woman on the other end of the telephone explains that she is Mrs. Grey and is calling about her husband who is in terrible pain. Indeed, in the background you can hear a man bellowing and moaning in pain. She says that he is too sick to come to the phone and then tells you this story: Her husband is 54 years old and began to have pain in the middle of his stomach about ten days ago. Four days ago it got worse, and she took him to another hospital's emergency department where the doctor took off his shirt and examined him, even ordered an upper GI x-ray series that was done and was normal. The doctor diagnosed "stomach flu" and sent him home with some Pepto-Bismol. Despite that therapy his pain had not remitted, and she now thought he was going to die if something was not done soon. You agree that he sounds pretty bad off and transfer the phone to your ambulance section so he can be picked up and brought in.

When he arrives at the ED half an hour later, an orderly undresses him and comes out to tell you the diagnosis. The orderly has noticed a swelling in the man's scrotum, mostly on the left side, that is, according to the orderly, melon sized. You go to see your patient and find that although he says his pain is periumbilical, the scrotal mass is very tender, not reducible, and refers pain or palpation to the middle of his abdomen. He tells you that the doctor at the other ED loosened his belt but never removed his pants during the examination four days ago. You diagnose an incarcerated inguinal hernia and call for a surgeon who takes your patient off to the operating room and solves the problem.

What is "stomach flu"?

What must the physical examination contain when the patient has pain in his mid abdomen?

What is "keyhole medicine"?

DISCUSSION   Influenza is, of course, an epidemic respiratory disease caused by a virus. It often appears in the winter and causes a self-limited illness with fever, cough, malaise, and other respiratory symptoms in young people but may be the last illness for older or chronically ill people. The lay public may refer to just about any sort of illness as "flu" and have extended the term to acute gastroenteritis by calling it "stomach flu." If we are to treat that lay term as even slightly specific, we ought to limit it to presumed viral infections lasting no more than a few days and presenting with nausea, vomiting, diarrhea, and weakness. We surely ought to be very careful applying such a term to any illness wherein abdominal pain is a cardinal symptom. Pain is often a symptom of serious intra-abdominal catastrophe and should be taken much more seriously.

Because of lack of time, we seldom can do as thorough a physical examination as we would like on many of our ED patients. But whatever we do, we must pay careful attention to vital signs. And we must examine the area of the body that the patient is complaining of. We must undress him and be sure that we consider what is connected to what. For example, a respiratory complaint should lead to a careful examination of the neck, the chest, and the entire circulatory system. An abdominal complaint should lead to examination not just of the abdomen but also of the chest, genitalia, pelvis, and rectum. Zachary Cope's dictum, "Semper per rectum," should not be forgotten. If we are rushed for time, we can be sure that there is not enough time to do the job badly and never enough time to warrant wasting it in "keyhole examinations" through partly unbuttoned or party removed clothing. Take it off, take it all off. You are not likely to miss a coconut in the scrotum if you uncover it and look at it. Again to quote Zachary Cope, "More harm is done by those who do not look, than by those who do not know what is in the book."

REFERENCES
Textbook   Tintinalli. Pp. 121–125.

Review Article   Nyhus, L. M., and Bombeck, C. T. Hernias. In D. C. Sabiston (ed.), *Textbook of Surgery*. Philadelphia, Saunders, 1986. Pp. 1231–1252.

Additional References   Janzon, L., Ryden, E. I., and Zederfeldt, B. Acute abdomen in surgical emergency room: Who is taking care of when for what? *Acta Chir. Scand.* 1982;148:141–148.

Zeta (Zachary Cope): *The Acute Abdomen In Verse.* London, H. K. Louis, 1962.

Case 12 Left Lower Quadrant Pain

A 35-year-old woman came to the emergency department complaining of low abdominal pain. The pain was bilateral but more marked on her left side. It had begun gradually the previous day and was not affected by anything she did. She denied having dysuria, changes in her bowel habits, vaginal discharge, or vaginal bleeding except for a few spots of blood on her pants the day before the pain began. She was ten days late for her period but had been slightly irregular in the past. She denied previous gynecologic problems.

On arrival she did not appear to be in any significant distress. She had normal respirations at a rate of 16, a pulse of 80, and a blood pressure of 120/80. Her abdomen had normal bowel sounds and was soft and nontender. There was no costovertebral angle tenderness. On pelvic examination she was found to have a normal parous cervix without any blood or discharge. Specimens of cervical mucus were obtained for chlamydia and gonorrhea cultures. She had a full, nontender bladder, mild cervical motion tenderness, and a moderately tender left adnexal region. The rectovaginal exam was normal and she had guiac negative stool.

The physician asked her to give a clean-catch urine sample and ordered a complete blood count (CBC) and a serum beta–human chorionic gonadotropin (beta-HCG) pregnancy test. The patient walked to the bathroom and was found five minutes later crouched at the bathroom door, holding on to the door jamb, appearing about to collapse.

Her nurse and doctor lifted her onto a stretcher and noted that she was then diaphoretic and had a pulse of 100 and a blood pressure of 80/50. They started two large-bore intravenous lines with lactated Ringer's solution and opened the stopcocks fully. They noted that her abdomen was more tender than it had been before, even to light palpation, and that bowel sounds were absent. A gynecologist was called and the operating room alerted. Her laparotomy began twenty minutes after her collapse. In the operating room, she was found to have

2000 ml of blood in the peritoneal cavity and a ruptured left tubal pregnancy.

What should be done when the diagnosis of ectopic pregnancy is first thought of?

What was there about her initial presentation that should have set off flashing lights in those caring for this healthy-looking patient?

DISCUSSION Ectopic pregnancy is often difficult to diagnose, but it is increasingly common. The possibility of this diagnosis should spring to mind in any young woman presenting with lateralized low abdominal pain. Patients with this condition often deteriorate abruptly.

This woman had lower abdominal pain, vaginal bleeding, a late period, and pain on adnexal palpation, all suggesting ectopic pregnancy; however, her differential diagnoses included salpingitis, ovarian cyst, appendicitis, and threatened abortion. After the history and physical exam, the first task in evaluating a woman with low abdominal pain of unknown origin is to determine whether or not she is pregnant.

This is not the first patient whose ectopic pregnancy ruptured after pelvic exam. Any patient whose history and physical suggest an ectopic pregnancy should be under observation with an intravenous line in place until the serum beta-HCG is known to be negative. If a urine specimen had been obtained prior to the examination, a urinary tract infection could have been ruled out and the bladder would have been empty, allowing a more accurate pelvic exam. A urine beta-HCG could have been done then. Some EDs do not have 24-hour access to serum tests for pregnancy and must rely on urine tests for HCG. Ectopic pregnancies generate lower levels of HCG than do intrauterine pregnancies, and occasionally the urine will be falsely negative.

If this patient had not worsened so dramatically and if an HCG was positive, then a pelvic ultrasound would have been ordered. If the ultrasound failed to show an intrauterine pregnancy, then she would have been admitted to the hospital for observation, serial HCG levels, and a repeat of the ultrasound. If this patient had arrived already in shock, rapid fluid resuscitation and immediate transfer to the operating room would have followed after a brief history and physical examination, intravenous line placement, and blood drawing for CBC, HCG, and crossmatching.

REFERENCES
Textbook   Rosen. Pp. 1591–1603.

Review Article   Hockberger, R. S. Ectopic pregnancy. *Emerg. Med. Clin. North Am.* 1987;5:481–493.

Additional References   Gennis, P., et al. Cost effectiveness of an accurate and rapid assay for serum human chorionic gonadotropin in suspected ectopic pregnancy. *Am. J. Emerg. Med.* 1988;6:4–6.

Patrick, J. D. Ectopic pregnancy—A brief review. *Ann. Emerg. Med.* 1982;11:576–581.

Abbott, J., et al. Ectopic pregnancy: Ten common pitfalls in diagnosis. *Am. J. Emerg. Med.* 1990;8:515–522.

Case 13 Drowned Child

The local rescue squad arrived at the emergency department ambulance ramp with a 16-year-old who had fallen into a nearby pond while ice-fishing with his father. The rescue worker said that it had taken them thirty-five minutes to retrieve him and that he was pulseless and apneic at the scene. Basic life support cardiopulmonary resuscitation efforts were begun immediately. He was ventilated using an esophageal-obturator airway (EOA).

At the ED, the boy was deeply cyanotic, cold, and without vital signs. His core body temperature was 28°C (83°F). His pupils were fixed and dilated.

Is there any point to going any further in this resuscitation?

What factors determine good outcome after prolonged submersion?

What is the esophageal-obturator airway?

DISCUSSION   The longest documented submersion with full neurologic recovery occurred in a 2½-year-old girl who was submerged in ice water for sixty-six minutes. The factors that determine good or poor outcome after prolonged submersion in ice water are still unclear. The "mammalian dive reflex" has been credited as a mechanism, but no substantial evidence supports this hypothesis. The shunting of blood from other parts of the body to the heart and brain that occurs in seals and other diving animals has never been shown to be of any significance in humans. Protection of the brain by decreasing its metabolic needs for oxygen through the development of acute submersion hypothermia is a more plausible explanation.

Regardless of the protective mechanism, the implication is that prolonged and heroic resuscitation attempts after submersion in very cold water are of value. Anyone profoundly hypothermic should not be declared dead until they are rewarmed, hence, the old dictum, "You are not dead until you are warm and dead."

The most important aspect of prehospital care is the immediate initiation of ventilation and oxygenation. Evidence of trauma should be noted and cervical spine precautions taken if indicated. Contributing factors such as hypoglycemia, seizures, and child neglect or abuse need to be considered. There is no logic in attempting to drain water from the lungs in fresh water drowning since the hypotonic fluid is rapidly absorbed. The Heimlich maneuver should not be performed unless there is inability to ventilate the patient due to an obstructed airway. Pushing on the stomach only increases the potential for emesis and aspiration of gastric contents.

In the ED critical patients should be intubated (going around the EOA, if necessary) and then hyperventilated. Continuous ECG and core temperature monitoring are needed. External rewarming modalities such as applying hot towels or heating lamps to the skin should be avoided since they produce peripheral vasodilation, allowing more cold, acidotic blood to enter the central circulation. The optimum rewarming method is extracorporeal blood rewarming combining a heart bypass machine with a heat exchanger. When extracorporeal rewarming is unavailable, peritoneal, gastric, bladder, or thoracic cavity lavage can be performed. Normal saline warmed to 106°F can be used as the irrigating solution.

The two most common complications manifest in near-drowning victims are cerebral and pulmonary edema. Cerebral edema is often managed with hyperventilation, fluid restriction, and diuretics. Positive end-expiratory pressure via assisted ventilation has been effective for the treatment of pulmonary edema.

The EOA is still used frequently in the prehospital setting. It is designed to be inserted down the throat and to occlude the esophagus, thus decreasing the likelihood of aspiration and allowing more effective bag-mask ventilation. Unfortunately, many complications are associated with its use, including accidental insertion down and occlusion of the airway, thus ensuring ventilation of the stomach!

REFERENCES

Textbook   Rosen. Pp. 645–651, 663–692.

Review Article   Martin, T. G. Neardrowning and cold water immersion. *Ann. Emerg. Med.* 1984;13:263–273.

Additional References   Neal, J. M. Near-drowning. *J. Emerg. Med.* 1985;3:41–52.

Bolte, R. G., et al. The use of extracorporeal rewarming in a child submerged for 66 minutes. *J.A.M.A.* 1988;260:377–379.

Case 14 An Otherwise Well Infant

A young monther came running into the emergency department with her 4-month-old infant son, screaming, "He's not breathing; he's not breathing."

The infant was cool, cyanotic, and without detectable pulse or blood pressure. He was intubated orally with a 3.5-mm endotracheal tube and was ventilated by bag as cardiac compression was begun. While efforts were made to start an intravenous line, 0.1 mg of epinephrine (1.0 ml of 1/10,000 solution) was given down the endotracheal tube and an intraosseous line was placed in the anterior tibia for administration of medications and fluids. Despite thirty minutes of resuscitative efforts, there was no evidence of cardiac response, and he was pronounced dead.

His mother said that he had been well, had eaten a good supper of formula and cereal, and went to bed uneventfully. He had a little nasal congestion the prior week but otherwise was well. She remembered that once, about a month earlier, she had gone to look at him sleeping and thought that he was not breathing. She touched him and he woke, crying, much to her relief. She had told her husband but he thought she was "just being a nervous mother."

The chaplain and a social worker were called to help console the family.

What is the most likely diagnosis?

What other diagnostic possibilities should be considered?

What is the primary event in pediatric cardiopulmonary arrest?

DISCUSSION   This is a classic presentation of sudden infant death syndrome (SIDS), commonly called "crib death." These infants are usually healthy and then suffer an unexpected cardiac and respiratory arrest. They are under 1 year of age, with the peak incidence at 2 to 4 months. The autopsy usually fails to define a cause of death. SIDS occurs more in fall and winter months, and sometimes the death is preceded by a mild respiratory infection. There may be a familial association with sleep apnea or periodic breathing. SIDS seems to occur more in lower socioeconomic families, and boys are at greater risk than girls. Infants of low birth weight and those with cigarette-smoking mothers are also at increased risk.

The cause of SIDS is unknown. Over seventy theories have been proposed, and the most accepted one suggests chronic hypoventilation and abnormal breathing reflexes secondary to an immature brain stem that predisposes the child to apnea and respiratory arrest.

One must consider trauma (child abuse), infections of the respiratory tract or the central nervous system, and congenital cardiac or metabolic defects. Seizures, intoxications, and botulism should also be considered.

Pediatric arrests differ from adult arrests in that the primary event is usually respiratory rather than cardiac. After prolonged hypoxia, the heart rhythm deteriorates to a bradycardia, and then to asystole.

Therapy is usually unsuccessful. The attempts in this infant exemplify the usual difficulty establishing an intravenous line for medication administration. Once an airway has been established, generally using an endotracheal tube of the same diameter as the child's little finger, certain medications can be given down the tube: epinephrine, atropine, lidocaine, and Narcan. Intraosseous cannulation of the anterior tibea can be used to administer medications intravascularly.

Although this case is typical of SIDS, the most common other diagnosis to look for is nonaccidental trauma or child abuse. We must be aware of the possibility of child abuse, but that awareness should not keep us from empathetic support of bereaved parents. SIDS support groups exist throughout the country, and parents of a child with SIDS should probably be referred to one for counselling and support.

REFERENCES
Textbook   Tintinalli. Pp. 409–411.

Review Article   Kelly, D. H., and Shannon, D. C. Sudden infant death syn-
                      drome and near-sudden infant death syndrome: A review of
                      the literature, 1964–1982. *Pediatr. Clin. North Am.* 1982;
                      29:1241–1257.

Additional   Schwartz, P. J., et al. The sudden infant death syndrome. *Ann
References*   N.Y. Acad. Sci.* 1988;535.

                      Meny, R. G., et al. Sudden infant death and home monitors.
                      Am. J. Dis. Child. 1988;142:1037–1040.

                      Oren, J., et al. Identification of the high risk group for sudden
                      infant death syndrome among infants who are resuscitated
                      from sleep apnea. *Pediatrics* 1986;77:495–499.

Case 15 Before the Accident

An 18-year-old man came to the emergency department following an auto accident. His car had hit a tree, and his forehead hit the windshield, lacerating his right brow. Because of crowded conditions in the ED, he was seen only briefly by a nurse and then obliged to wait almost two hours before a physician could suture his wound. At the time of treatment, he claimed he felt fine, although he had been rather tired while waiting and appreciated the chance to rest. A cursory neurologic examination revealed no abnormalities. His laceration was debrided, cleaned, and sutured with 5-0 nylon. His eyebrow was not shaved. Because his last tetanus toxoid had been at age 8, he was given 0.5 ml of tetanus toxoid. The sutures were removed four days later, and his wound had healed well.

Four months later the man returned to the ED in the company of his mother. She claimed that he had been passing out since his injury. He had had about six episodes during which he stopped all activity, stared at the floor for several minutes, and once or twice fell to the floor. There were no associated involuntary movements and no incontinence. On close questioning, the patient recalled having a few spells during the year preceding his auto accident. He could not recall the exact events of his accident and never had been aware of striking the tree. After a faint, he usually would be a bit fatigued and sometimes momentarily confused. He denied dizziness, headache, or other symptoms. A thorough neurologic examination showed nothing abnormal, and there was no change of pulse or blood pressure when he changed from recumbent to standing position.

What is the matter with this young man?

Was his initial therapy correct?

What studies should be done?

DISCUSSION   The situation surrounding an accident may be of more importance than the event itself. It is possible that a more prompt
physician evaluation of the young man described here might
have revealed significant confusion and lethargy, pointing to
preexisting neurologic disease or concussion. The past history
regarding lapses of consciousness is pertinent. In any case, the
subsequent ED visit suggests that the patient is having recurrent
losses of consciousness and that a seizure disorder may be present. An EEG and computed tomography scan would be appropriate, and he deserves a followup evaluation by a neurologist.
You should always consider these four possible "S" causes of
single car accidents: seizure, syncope, sugar (low), and suicide;
as well as the two most common "S" causes, sleep and sauce
(booze).

The patient's initial evaluation should have included a thorough neurologic examination (not the cursory one noted in the
case). If his neurologic examination (including a mental status
exam) was in any way abnormal, a computed tomography scan
of the head would have been ordered at that time to rule out an
intracranial bleed (subdural or epidural hematoma) or a contusion of the brain. Patients with these injuries require admission
and neurosurgical monitoring. On the initial visit, the patient
should also have had an evaluation for cervical spine injury,
since cervical-spine injury should always be suspected in anyone having any head injury. It is occasionally possible to "clinically" (without x-ray) rule out cervical spine fractures in a fully
alert patient if there is no neck pain or tenderness and no pain on
neck movement. Generally, x-rays are needed if the patient is
symptomatic or has a mental status that is in any way abnormal.

The initial treatment of this patient's laceration was correct.
Most authorities believe that eyebrows may not be shaved with
impunity. If shaved, the eyebrow may not grow back normally.
If no tetanus toxoid had ever been given to the patient, he
would have been given 250 units of human tetanus immune
globulin followed by a tetanus toxoid immunization program.
When a patient has received tetanus immunization within the
last ten years, a booster dose of toxoid will call forth an adequate amnestic response.

The repair of facial lacerations such as this young man's
should be done as quickly as possible after the injury, but,
because of the excellent blood supply, the face may be primarily closed as long as eighteen hours after the injury. Wound
preparation should be preceded by adequate local anesthesia,
generally with lidocaine (Xylocaine). If using an epinephrine-

containing mixture, this provides hemostasis as well as anesthesia and can be used on most areas of the face except the ears, tip of nose, and lips. The wound should be thoroughly cleaned and sutured with minimal if any debridement. Deep muscle and subcuticular tissues should be approximated with 5-0 Dexon sutures. The skin should be closed with fine nonabsorbable sutures such as 6-0 nylon. A plastic surgeon should generally be consulted if there is a large facial laceration with tissue loss or if there is a concern about the cosmetic result on the part of the patient or the physician.

REFERENCES

Textbook   Rosen. Pp. 363–373, 388–392.

Review Article   Long, C. J., and Novack, T. A. Symptoms after head trauma. *South. Med. J.* 1986;79:728–732.

Additional   Dushoff, I. M. About face (principles of wound repair). *Emerg.*
Reference   *Med.* November 1974;6:24–77.

An 18-year-old woman was brought into the emergency department in a wheelchair. She had been assisted from a car and into the chair, but by the end of her 100-foot ride into the ED, she had stopped breathing and her color was blue-gray. A pulse was present, although thready, at a rate of about 80. She was lifted onto a bed and began to vomit thin, green liquid. Her head was turned to the side and her pharynx suctioned with a rigid (Yankauer) sucker. An oral airway was placed, and her lungs were ventilated with a self-inflating bag for about a minute while one of the doctors readied an endotracheal tube and a laryngoscope. When he was ready, the bag was removed and he succeeded in placing an oral tube in her trachea within one minute. If it had taken over one minute, the resuscitation chief would have terminated the attempt and returned to the Ambu bag.

A nurse spoke with the patient's friend who had brought her to the ED and obtained information that the patient might have taken an overdose of propoxyphene (Darvon). A 2-mg dose of Narcon was given intravenously. The patient had a minor motor seizure involving face and arms lasting one to two minutes. An intravenous infusion of 5% dextrose in water was started. Four more brief seizures followed. Ventilation continued with a self-inflating bag attached to the endotracheal tube, and another 2-mg dose of Narcan was given intravenously ten minutes after the first dose. The patient's breathing returned, and her color improved. A Foley catheter was placed in her bladder, and 300 ml of urine was sent to the lab for toxicology study. A blood sample was drawn (with H_2O_2 rather than isopropyl alcohol used to scrub the skin) and sent to the laboratory for alcohol, barbiturate, glucose, BUN, and electrolyte analyses, and for CBC. A portable chest film was obtained, and a brief examination was made for neurologic and other major abnormalities. An esophageal tube (large bore, Ewald type) was placed in the stomach, and the patient was lavaged with 2000 ml of tap water in 400-ml amounts. The endotracheal tube cuff was inflated during all these events.

The patient was transferred to the medical intensive care unit within one hour of her arrival at the ED. While she was being transferred to a cart for the trip to the intensive care unit, a marijuana cigarette fell out of her jacket pocket. She awoke six hours later and admitted to taking about sixty Darvon capsules.

Her ED visit required the attention of three physicians and two nurses.

What are the most urgent activities in an overdose case such as this?

What do the seizures suggest?

Was the Narcan the only therapeutic maneuver responsible for her improvement?

DISCUSSION   Amazingly, a fair number of patients seem to make it to the door of the ED and expire there. This patient was clearly dying on arrival. Only rapid, vigorous, knowledgeable, and well-coordinated care could help her. A ten-minute delay would have been fatal.

This patient arrived in acute brain and respiratory failure. The only appropriate therapy was to secure control of her airway and ventilate her. The airway is best controlled via an endotracheal tube, and a self-inflating bag is best for ventilation.

Emesis with aspiration is an ever-present danger during resuscitation and can be adequately guarded against only by obstructing the trachea with a cuffed tube. Intubation will take seconds to minutes, and ventilation usually should be obtained first with a face mask. Before attempting intubation, the physician must ready all equipment: laryngoscope, endotracheal tube and stylet, lubricant, syringe to inflate the cuff, suction, and connectors for attachment of the tube to the source of ventilation, such as a self-inflating bag. The intubator should try holding his or her breath while attempting intubation. When the intubator needs to breathe, the patient should be hyperventilated using a bag with a mask.

Intravenous access should always be established. This may prove difficult in intravenous drug abusers, and if no simple percutaneous access is available, a cutdown should be performed or a central line established. Any patient in coma from an unknown cause, including suspected drug overdoses, should be given an intravenous "cocktail" of 50 cc of 50% glucose solution and at least two 0.4 mg amps of naloxone (Narcan). Both are almost entirely safe and can cause a rapid cure for coma from hypoglycemia and narcotics, respectively. Larger doses of either can be used if required. Most centers with a high proportion of chronic alcoholic patients routinely give 50 or 100 mg of thiamine also.

Seizures in an overdose patient are often the result of hypoxia. Certain drugs are notorious for causing seizures, even in the absence of hypoxia. These include Darvon, meperidine, antidepressants, theophylline, INH, cocaine and other sympathomimetics, anticholinergics, and antihistamines.

Naloxone (Narcan) is very effective in reversing narcotics overdose effects. It is less effective against Darvon than against heroin but still often is helpful. When treating patients with narcotics overdoses, one must be aware that the duration of action of heroin or other narcotics is far greater than the duration of action of any available narcotic antagonist. A patient may wake up, pull out the endotracheal tube, talk to the attendant, perhaps even be discharged, and then return to coma and hypoventilation as the antagonist wears off.

Any patient who has become hypoxic will be more obtunded than warranted by just the central nervous system depressive effect of the overdose drug. We have found that such patients respond well to ventilation for five to ten minutes. Thus, ventilation alone may return the patient to a state where she can adequately carry on ventilation thereafter. This may make the effect of the narcotic antagonist harder to evaluate.

The evaluation of this patient's overdose should also include an acetaminophen level since she could have taken a combination drug such as Darvocet or, as frequently happens, taken other pills the providers were unaware of. Treatment can be begun early in the course of the case if it is suspected that the patient took a toxic dose of acetaminophen. N-acetylcysteine (Mucomyst) given orally is the antidote. Acetaminophen overdose is initially asymptomatic but can produce fulminant and fatal hepatic failure days later if not treated.

REFERENCES

Textbook   Rosen. Pp. 2125–2138.

Review Article   Handal, K. A., Schauben, J. L., and Salamone, F. R. Naloxone. *Ann. Emerg. Med.* 1983;12:438–445.

Additional Reference   Allbutt, C. On the abuse of hypodermic injections of morphine. *Practitioner* 1870;5:327–331.

Case 17 Honking Horn on the Ambulance Ramp

A 55-year-old man was brought to the ambulance ramp in a car by his wife. She remained in her car and honked its horn continuously. Several seconds later a clerk, an aide, and two nurses ran out with a stretcher. They found the patient drenched in sweat, unable to speak, and leaning forward in his seat. His wife started screaming, "He can't breathe, he can't breathe, do something."

The patient was immediately brought to a treatment area where he was attached to a cardiac monitor and placed on a nonrebreathing mask to deliver 100% oxygen. He kept pulling the oxygen mask off. An intravenous line of 5% dextrose in water was established. His blood pressure was 170/90, pulse 80, and respirations 36 per minute.

Examination revealed coarse rales throughout both lung fields, and the respiratory noise obscured his heart tones. Sitting up, his neck veins were distended to the angle of the jaw, and there was slight pitting pretibial edema. He was very agitated and his skin was cool and very diaphoretic. He nodded when asked about chest pain but was unable to speak. He preferred to sit bolt upright and to lean slightly forward. Morphine sulfate 2 mg and furosemide 40 mg were given intravenously, and one nitroglycerin tablet 1/150 grain (0.4 mg) was given sublingually.

His wife said that her husband had a "mild" heart attack about two years earlier and had hypertension. He also was under a doctor's care for an irregular heart rhythm, but his only medications were hydrochlorothiazide and propranolol. He told her that he had been feeling a little short of breath with exertion over the past few days and had complained of chest pain about an hour before the acute onset of shortness of breath.

What are the priorities in treating acute pulmonary edema?

What further evaluation is needed in assessment and treatment of these patients?

DISCUSSION   The patient presented in acute respiratory failure due to acute
pulmonary edema. This is most often due to cardiac decom-
pensation and left ventricular failure but can also be from noncardiac causes such as smoke inhalation, near drowning, high
altitude, trauma, pneumonia, aspiration, and heroin overdose.
Optimally, a patient like this gets highly sophisticated advanced
life support provided by paramedics in an ambulance, and
luckily for all of us, this type of care is increasingly common. In
this case, he was brought in a car by his wife. She was hysterical because she recognized the severity of his condition and was
concerned for his life. On arriving at the emergency department, she used the car horn to summon assistance. Well-sea-
soned ED staff members are always alert to unusual commo-
tions outside the doors of the department. Patients will
frequently present in this manner.

One can gauge the intensity of this patient's respiratory distress by his inability to speak. He was expending all his energy
to breathe. The typical presentation of these patients is in the
sitting position. This maximizes their ability to breathe by using
gravity to aid diaphragmatic excursions. Lung sounds will usually be very noisy with rales present throughout the lung fields.
There may be wheezes present due to airway spasm and
edema ("cardiac asthma"). The blood pressure is frequently
elevated, and there is usually tachycardia. Patients on beta-
blockers may have normal heart rates since the usual sympathetic response is blocked. The heart sounds are usually inaud-
ible because of the noisy lungs, but, if audible, S_3 and S_4 gallops may be present. The skin is usually cool and moist,
reflecting decreased cutaneous perfusion. If the cardiac output
is severely depressed, cyanosis and hypotension may be present. These are ominous signs. Pedal edema and jugular venous
pressure elevation are signs of accompanying right heart failure,
but they are not always present.

The immediate concern of the ED staff is to begin treatment
and prevent complications such as hypoxia-mediated myocardial infarction or arrest. The initial treatment is high-flow oxygen delivered by a face mask with a reservoir bag attached.
The patient is placed on a cardiac monitor and an intravenous
line is established. The solution of choice is 5% dextrose in
water since salt will make the heart failure worse. Furosemide
and morphine sulfate are given intravenously as soon as possible. Furosemide is a mild venodilator and potent diuretic. Morphine is a sedative and a venodilator. Because of their hypoxia,
these patients will be very anxious and may refuse to keep an

oxygen mask in place. Providing a small amount of sedation will reduce the work of the heart. Nitroglycerin will dilate veins and arteries and should initially be given in the sublingual form. It is a rapidly acting treatment for pulmonary edema and is especially helpful in the patient who is experiencing some coronary ischemia and having chest pain with the episode. In the prehospital area, paramedics can begin much of this treatment including the use of oxygen, nitroglycerin, furosemide, and in some areas morphine sulfate. Rotating venous constricting bands (incorrectly called rotating tourniquets) were frequently used in the past. They are still sometimes used as an adjunct measure in severe cases.

After the initial therapy has been begun, the patient's response can be judged by following his vital signs and ability to speak. If his pulse decreases and he is able to speak a few words, the process may be improving. In very severe cases, the therapy mentioned above is either not sufficient or too late. A prompt decision to nasotracheally intubate frequently saves lives in this setting.

Very few laboratory tests will be useful in the acute management of this patient. A portable chest x-ray is required to show the degree of edema, although the patient's clinical improvement will precede the improvement on the x-ray. A complete blood count should be obtained (to look for anemia), as should baseline electrolytes, BUN, glucose, creatinine, and cardiac enzymes. An ECG should be obtained initially and repeated when the patient is more comfortable and has a slower heart rate. This may show signs of ischemia. None of these tests, neither the obtaining nor the interpretation of them, ever takes precedence over ensuring adequate ventilation.

A number of other pharmacologic interventions may help these patients. Beta-blockers are contraindicated in patients with heart failure and should be cut back immediately if a patient on them develops heart failure. Aminophylline can be given if there is a large component of bronchospasm. Arrhythmias should be treated as needed (ventricular arrhythmias with lidocaine or countershock, and supraventricular arrhythmias with verapamil or countershock). Digitalis preparations were widely used in the past but are less used now in the treatment of acute pulmonary edema. They are used to treat supraventricular tachycardia due to atrial fibrillation. These patients will almost invariably require admission to the coronary care unit since an acute myocardial infarction cannot be ruled out.

Occasionally patients will present early in the course of worsening heart failure. The early symptoms are increasing shortness of breath, paroxysmal nocturnal dyspnea, and orthopnea. These are not always present or the patient may not be aware of the significance of the sensations. Your interviewing style may help the patient correctly identify these symptoms. The patient should be asked about his level of exercise and if there was any recent change. Other useful questions include the number of pillows used at night; change in sleep patterns, especially midnight or early morning wakening; new onset of coughing, light-headedness; nausea; or changes in appetite. Commonly, a patient may have consumed an unusually large amount of salt in his diet, or forgotten to take his medication. The sudden worsening of heart failure can signal myocardial ischemia or infarction even without the presence of chest pain.

REFERENCES

Textbook   Rosen. Pp. 1291–1301.

Review Article   Ruggie, E. N. Congestive heart failure. *Med. Clin. North Am.* 1986;70:829–841..

Additional Reference   Robin, E. D., Closs, C. E., and Zellis, R. Pulmonary edema. *N. Engl. J. Med.* 1973;288:229–246, 292–304.

Case 18 Monoarticular Arthritis

A 30-year-old man came to the emergency department at 2 A.M. complaining of pain and swelling in his left knee for several hours. He had previously been well, although on careful questioning he admitted to having had some burning on urination for a few days about two weeks earlier. He recalled no trauma to the knee and was on no medications.

Physical examination revealed that the patient had a warm, slightly erythematous, swollen left knee. The knee was tender, and attempts at flexion led to severe pain. All his other joints seemed normal. His conjunctiva were normal, and he had no urethral discharge. He had no heart murmur, no skin rash, no adenopathy, and no hepatosplenomegaly. He had no nodules, tophi, or other lumps and was afebrile.

He was given codeine for his pain and referred to the arthritis clinic in two days.

Is acute monarticular arthritis ever an emergency?

Would you advise any laboratory studies?

Is there any danger in handling this case in this fashion?

DISCUSSION   There are few true rheumatologic emergencies. An acute non-traumatic monarticular arthritis is one of these. If the patient has not traumatized the joint by twisting, falling, or hitting it, and if he is not on anticoagulants or a known bleeder, then two common causes of an acute monarticular arthritis should be suspected: acute gout or a septic joint. Either one may be excruciatingly painful, but the grave danger lies in missing the diagnosis of a bacterial arthritis. A septic joint may be destroyed within forty-eight hours, hence rapid diagnosis and initiation of correct therapy are required.

The diagnostic procedure is a joint aspiration. It is quite easy to tap the knee medially under the patella if there is any effusion. Sterile technique should be used with care to avoid introducing bacteria into a previously sterile joint. The aspirate should be cultured, a sample should be placed in a heparinized tube to examine for crystals, a white blood cell count should be done with saline solution as a diluent, and a gram stain of a smear should be made. If the white cell count is attempted with the usual acetic acid diluent, the cells will clump in the precipitated mucus and the count will be falsely low. Someone experienced at looking for crystals should use a polarized light microscope to search for uric acid or the calcium pyrophosphate crystals seen in pseudogout. Cultures should be carefully done and should include a specific culture medium for gonococcus. When evidence of gout or pseudogout is lacking, treatment for sepsis should be initiated without waiting for culture results if the joint leukocyte count is high.

Gonococcal arthritis should be suspected in any sexually active person who presents with a single hot joint. Skin pustules on a purplish or erythematous base may be present, and one may be able to aspirate gonococci (for culture or gram stain) from these lesions.

A patient with a septic joint urgently needs hospitalization. Even if the correct diagnosis is gout, the patient deserves more rapid diagnosis and therapy than were given in this case. Most patients who come to the ED at 2 A.M. are in significant distress, and they deserve rapid, effective care.

On arrival at the rheumatology clinic two days after his ED visit, this man's knee was tapped. The aspirated fluid had a white cell count of 15,500 per cu mm, and uric acid crystals were seen in some of the leukocytes. His acute attack was subsiding, and followup care was arranged.

Acute gout may be best treated acutely with colchicine (0.5 mg hourly by mouth) until the joint improves or diarrhea ap-

pears—they usually occur simultaneously—or with indo-
methacin (50 mg qid for one day and 25 mg qid for subsequent
days) or with another nonsteroidal anti-inflammatory agent, in
adequate (large) doses. Before therapy is begun, the patient
should have a CBC, blood uric acid, and rheumatoid preparation. The joint should be x-rayed, and followup should be arranged.

REFERENCES
Textbook   Rosen. Pp. 832–833, 892.

Review Article   Smith, J. W. Infectious Arthritis. In G. L. Mandell, R. G. Dou-
                           glas, J. E. Bennett (eds.), *Principles and Practice of Infectious
                           Diseases*, 2nd edition. New York, Churchill Livingstone,
                           1985. Pp. 697–704.

Additional   Sternbach, G. L., and Baker, F. J. Emergency joint arthrocen-
Reference   tesis and synovial fluid analysis. *JACEP* 1976;5:787–792.

Case **19** They Had Never Seen Anything Like It Before

A 64-year-old man was brought to the emergency department at 8 P.M. by his wife because of her concern that his scrotum was swollen and tender. He was not too eager to obtain medical care and volunteered little history but claimed to have been well previously and to have had scrotal swelling for about two days. He had chilling but had not taken his temperature. He was not on any medications and emphatically did not wish to remain in the hospital as an inpatient.

On examination, the patient appeared slightly confused and irritable but in no other distress. His temperature was 38.8°C orally, pulse 110, respiration 18, and blood pressure 150/90. His scrotum was swollen, slightly edematous, tender throughout, and erythematous. There was no remarkable inguinal lymphadenopathy. The scrotum was so tender as to prevent careful palpation.

The patient was seen by a medical resident, who admitted that the problem looked like some sort of an infection but that he had never seen anything quite like it before. The man was also seen by a urology resident, who admitted that he too had never seen such a problem before. They elected to treat him with rest and oral antibiotics.

Two days later the patient had deteriorated further and was brought back to the ED by his wife. He was more obtunded and even less communicative than before. His scrotum was further swollen and darker in color—almost black in areas—and swelling extended up the thighs and lower abdomen. Slight crepitus in the scrotum was noted.

This time the man was admitted to the hospital, and initial laboratory studies indicated he was in diabetic ketoacidosis. Major surgical debridement of the scrotum was done in the operating room. His subsequent hospital course was very stormy, with an episode of acute renal failure.

What diseases predispose to bizarre infection?

What simple laboratory tests can be done in the ED to look

63

for these predisposing disorders?

What organisms are most commonly responsible for gas gangrene?

DISCUSSION Remarkable diseases should be remarked on. This case puzzled both the medical and the urologic consultants, yet they were content to treat him as an example of a less bizarre illness and obtained no laboratory studies to search for other underlying diseases. The patient paid a price for this error in judgment.

A major red flag in this case was that the patient presented with abnormal vital signs. The presence of fever over 101°F (38.3°C) in a person over the age of 60 is more worrisome and more likely to herald serious underlying infection than in younger persons. This man also had another clinical sign experienced clinicians rarely ignore: a resting tachycardia. Any abnormal vital sign must be investigated thoroughly, and a resting tachycardia is often the premonitory sign of an impending disaster.

Additionally, an altered mental status should always prompt a detailed investigation for an underlying cause. This man presented with slight confusion and irritability. A mental status examination should be performed on a patient exhibiting altered behavior. Clues to an organic cause for the confusion include disorientation (person, place, time, or purpose) and inability to name common objects or perform simple subtraction of serial sevens. The acute onset of an organic brain syndrome should always prompt a search for a metabolic cause (hypoxia, acidosis, infection, electrolyte abnormality, or drug or other intoxication).

Hematologic disorders, diabetes mellitus, uremia, and immunodeficiency lead the list of diseases predisposing to unusual infections. A blood sugar, BUN, and CBC would have adequately screened for the first three and would have picked up the diabetes. Even a simple urinalysis would have led to detection of the ketoacidosis. Missing this ancillary diagnosis surely allowed the infection to remain out of control despite antibiotic therapy.

Gas-forming bacteria are plentiful. The three most commonly seen are clostridia, bacteroids, and nonhemolytic streptococcus. Penicillin used with an aminoglycoside to cover for gram-negative infection is fine for antibiotic coverage, but third-generation cephalosporins can also be used. Surgical drainage and debridement are essential, as is control of such associated problems as ketoacidosis. Ketoacidosis is itself a serious disorder with a significant mortality. It is usually viewed as a medical emergency requiring hospitalization and urgent therapy.

REFERENCES
Textbook Tintinalli. Pp. 490–495.

Review Article   Kitabchi, A. E., and Murphy, M. B. Diabetic ketoacidosis and hyperglycemic nonketotic coma. *Med. Clin. North Am.* 1988;72:1545–1563.

Additional   Keating, H. J., et al. Effect age has on the clinical significance of
Reference   fever in ambulatory adult patients. *J. Am. Geriatr. Soc.* 1984;32:282–287.

Case 20 Asthma

A 23-year-old man was brought to the emergency department from the city jail one evening because he had become short-winded. He had suffered bronchial asthma since childhood and had been on corticosteroids in the past but not lately. His usual therapy consisted of oral bronchodilator tablets and an Isuprel inhaler. On the evening of his ED admission, he had been arrested for verbally abusing a police officer who was trying to get him to move his car from an illegal parking area at an outdoor rock music festival. While in jail, the man had become short of breath and begun to wheeze. His jailers had him taken to the ED.

On arrival he appeared in only minimal respiratory distress. He was afebrile and had bilateral musical wheezes in his chest. An occasional nonproductive cough was apparent. His vital signs were temperature 37.0°C, pulse 90, respiration 20, blood pressure 150/80.

Therapy was begun with oxygen by nasal prongs at a flow rate of 5 liters per minute, and an intravenous infusion of 500 mg of aminophylline in 500 ml of 5% dextrose solution was given over a two-hour period. At the end of this period, the patient felt better, his wheezes were "less tight," and he was returned to the city jail.

During the next six hours he became dyspneic again and used his pocket isoproterenol (Isuprel) inhaler frequently in his jail cell. He was then returned to the ED, where he was seen almost immediately by a physician. His vital signs now were temperature 37°C, pulse 110 and regular, respiration 22, blood pressure 154/82. His chest had diffuse wheezes but did seem to be ventilating adequately. He was not cyanotic. His heart sounded normal, and he had no edema. He was given 0.4 mg of epinephrine subcutaneously and within three minutes suffered a cardiac arrest. Despite vigorous immediate attempts at cardiopulmonary resuscitation, he could not be resuscitated.

Is epinephrine usually considered to be the drug of choice in treating asthma?

If this patient's death was not due purely to chance, what could have been the physiologic state due to asthma prior to the epinephrine injection that predisposed him to a fatal arrhythmia?

What other disorders can present in the ED as "asthma"?

DISCUSSION   Asthma is a serious disease that is increasingly associated with sudden death, especially in users of inhaled bronchodilator aerosols. Asthmatics may become either alkalotic or acidotic. Either of these may be injurious, but in the setting of hypoxia and sympathomimetic loading, acidosis is more dangerous. Acidotic hypoxic hearts are very vulnerable to arrhythmias when sympathomimetics are given. If a sympathomimetic must be given when the patient might be hypoxic, it may be best not to give it by intravenous push or intramuscular or subcutaneous injection. The physician caring for the patient may not have fully appreciated the patient's self-administered "bronchodilator" and the possibility of serious hypoxia and pH abnormality. Infrequent premature ventricular contractions may have been present but missed. Unlike isoproterenol and epinephrine, most modern inhaled bronchodilators have a selective beta-1 effect on the lungs without as much beta-2 effect on the heart. Metaproterenol (Metaprel) and albuterol (Ventolin) can be used in these patients with a higher degree of safety.

Only an asthmatic given no prior therapy, with several hours of dyspnea at most, who requests the drug because it worked best for him or her in the past, and with no notable fatigue now receives epinephrine in our ED. Pediatric asthma patients are somewhat different, and with them epinephrine may be less dangerous. Epinephrine is still usually considered an effective drug in asthma, but in a patient already loaded with sympathomimetics, the discomfort of the injection and the hazard of a fatal arrhythmia leads us to use other drugs.

There are many ways to treat asthma, and some variation from center to center. Our approach is to give oxygen nasally and then immediately give a nebulized bronchodilator treatment. Patients on theophylline should have a theophylline level drawn, and then, unless there is a question of an overdose, they should be started on a maintenance infusion of the drug. Patients not on theophylline can be given a loading dose over no less than twenty minutes and then placed on a maintenance infusion. The patient should be well hydrated to loosen secretions: a 400- or 500-ml bolus of fluid in a young patient is perfectly reasonable. Intravenous steroids should be initiated early in any patient who has been on steroids before. The peak expiratory flow rate is a useful measurement of the patient's response to therapy. An improvement should be seen after the first treatment and is a good sign. Patients not improving after the first treatment or whose peak flows are still below 300 liters per minute after three nebulized bronchodilator treatments should be considered for admission. If the patient has a fever, purulent-appearing sputum, or infiltrate on the chest x-ray, or fails to improve dramatically in six hours in the ED, he almost surely needs to be hospitalized.

Fatigue is very dangerous and argues for admission. Extreme fatigue is an indication for elective nasotracheal intubation. A skillfully inserted nasotracheal tube is usually well tolerated and a great relief to a tired asthmatic.

Some asthmatics are regularly harder to treat than others. One should suspect that the current case will be a difficult one when the patient relates a past use of steroids. Many very difficult cases of asthma are referred to special treatment centers, and a patient who has been so treated should be assumed to have asthma that does not respond easily to therapeutic efforts. The case described had such a history. Above all, the patient may be able to tell the doctor what therapy has been helpful or harmful to him in the past. Listen to him (of course, he may well ask for "a shot of adrenalin"). Asthma is seldom easy to deal with.

The diagnosis of asthma is not always correct. Most commonly, the middle-aged or older patient who comes in claiming that his "asthma is giving him trouble" is *not* an asthmatic but rather has an exacerbation of chronic bronchitis, emphysema, or heart failure. As usual, the key to correct therapy is correct diagnosis, and one must not accept the patient's own diagnosis as correct. Obviously a patient in heart failure with "cardiac asthma" should not be given large amounts of fluids intravenously. A careful initial appraisal should seek evidence of heart failure such as elevated venous pressure or edema.

REFERENCES
Textbook   Tintinalli. Pp. 275–282.

Review Articles   Brenner, B. E. Bronchial asthma in adults: Presentation to the emergency department, part 1: Pathogenesis, clinical manifestation, diagnostic evaluation, and differential diagnosis. *Am. J. Emerg. Med.* 1983;1:50–70.

Brenner, B. E. Bronchial asthma in adults: Presentation to the emergency department, part 2: Sympathomimetics, respiratory failure, recommendation for initial treatment, indication for admission, and summary. *Am. J. Emerg. Med.* 1983;3: 306–333.

Additional Reference

Schnieder, S. M. Effect of a treatment protocol on the efficiency of care of the adult acute asthmatic. *Ann. Emerg. Med.* 1986; 15:703–706.

Case 21 A Request for Methadone

A 21-year-old man came to the emergency department requesting a prescription for methadone. He stated that he was a heroin addict and used $200 to $300 worth of street heroin a day. He claimed heavy use of heroin for two years and heavy involvement in burglary to support his habit. Now he wished to stop taking the heroin and was feeling ill after having no drug for twelve hours.

On physical examination, no abnormalities were observed. The patient's veins were not scarred ("tracks"); he had no round subcutaneous dimples (results of "skin popping"); and his pupils were midposition and reactive to light. Blood pressure was 130/50, pulse 95, respiration 16, and temperature 37.0°C.

The patient was given 40 mg of methadone (in 10-mg tablets) and left the ED. Six hours later he was returned to the ED deeply comatose but with adequate respiration and blood pressure. A friend stated that the patient had taken the methadone "to get high," that he had *not* been on heroin, and had drunk some vodka. His blood alcohol was 346 mg per dl (also called "346 milligrams percent"). Narcan, 2 mg given intravenously, produced no notable change, and the patient was kept in the ED under observation for twelve hours to "sleep it off."

What are the signs and symptoms of heroin withdrawal?

If a presumed heroin addict has seizures during a withdrawal period, what was he likely taking?

Is methadone an innocuous drug?

DISCUSSION   This patient was obviously mainly drunk; however, the combination of methadone and alcohol is very dangerous, and the prescribing of methadone should be part of a maintenance program and not done in the ED unless enrollment in such a program can be proven and the dose verified by a supervisor at the program. This patient was probably neither a heroin addict nor withdrawing from heroin.

Diaphoresis, dilated pupils, rhinorrhea, diarrhea, and colicky abdominal pain are early signs of narcotics withdrawal. Evidence of injection sites—usually needle tracks on arm veins—should be sought. People with inadequate veins (including chronic users in whom all available veins have thrombosed) may resort to "skin popping" or subcutaneous injection. They are prone to local abscesses, cellulitis, hepatitis B, acquired immunodeficiency syndrome, tetanus, endocarditis, pneumonia, strokes, and lesser complications such as constipation, neuropathies, and secondary amenorrhea.

Seizures are not part of the narcotics withdrawal syndrome. Often street heroin or "horse" or "smack" is not truly heroin or contains only a small dose of heroin diluted with other drugs. Quinine, because it is white, powdery, bitter, and produces flushing when given intravenously, is often mixed with barbiturate (for narcosis) unbeknown to the addict. Such a drug might lead to heroin withdrawal symptoms in an addict and later to barbiturate withdrawal symptoms such as seizures.

In general, it is best to treat a patient for narcotics withdrawal only when signs of that state are apparent and then to give 10 to 20 mg a day of methadone or other narcotic in equivalent dose while keeping the patient under observation. This dosage can be given until the patient is less ill or gets into a maintenance program. This dosage will take the edge off true heroin withdrawal symptoms but will not harm a user who is exaggerating his habit. It will not be enough to totally relieve an addict who is used to large doses of narcotics; he will still feel ill, even if not as ill as he would on no drug at all.

Methadone is widely used in the United States in maintenance therapy for chronic heroin addicts to prevent heroin euphoria and withdrawal symptoms. In such a program, a tolerant addict is usually given a daily dose of 60 to 120 mg of methadone; although, to a nontolerant person, even 40 mg could be a very large dose. Mixed with alcohol or other sedatives, this amount of methadone can be fatal, acting as a respiratory depressant like any other narcotic.

In lieu of methodone and its problems in the acute setting,

clonidine can also be used for the treatment of addicts who are displaying symptoms of withdrawal.

REFERENCES

Textbook   Rosen. Pp. 2136–2138.

Review Article   Freitas, P. M. Narcotic withdrawal in the emergency depart-
                      ment. *Am. J. Emerg. Med.* 1985;3:456–460.

Additional   Kleber, H. D., and Riordan, C. E. The treatment of narcotic
Reference   withdrawal: A historical review. *J. Clin. Psychiatry*
                      1982;43:30–34.

Case 22 Twenty-Eight Year Old with Chest Pain

A 28-year-old man came to the emergency department one evening complaining of chest pain. He stated that the pain began about an hour earlier, was substernal and crushing in nature, and radiated into his left arm. He had never had any pain like this before and had not been exerting himself heavily before the pain began. He was a nonsmoker and did not drink alcohol to excess. There was no family history of diabetes, hypertension, or heart disease.

His blood pressure was 154/96, pulse 112, respirations 18, and he was afebrile. He appeared extremely anxious. His neck veins were flat while he was lying at 20 degrees. His lungs were clear and his heart tones were normal. The abdomen was benign without organomegaly and his legs were nontender without edema. His deep tendon reflexes were slightly hyperactive and he had a fine tremor. An ECG showed "early repolarization" but was otherwise within normal limits.

He was placed on a cardiac monitor, given oxygen by nasal prongs, and an intravenous line was started with 5% dextrose in water at a keep-open rate. A chest x-ray was normal. He was given sublingual nitroglycerin tablets for the pain. After three tablets had only decreased the pain from 10 to 3 on a scale of 10, he was given some morphine intravenously. This relieved his pain and allayed his anxiety.

Further history was obtained at this time. He admitted that he had just been at a party where he had some cocaine for the second time in his life. He had first tried cocaine several weeks earlier without any problem. That evening he had snorted two lines of cocaine and soon felt his heart pounding in his chest. The chest pain began shortly thereafter.

He was admitted to the coronary care unit where further workup showed that he had sustained a small anterior myocardial infarction. He was subsequently discharged without sequela.

What are the effects of cocaine use?

What are the priorities in the treatment of sympathomimetic overdose?

In cocaine abuse, how is the treatment of a "body packer" different from that of a "body stuffer"?

DISCUSSION   The typical presentation seen with a cocaine overdose is euphoria followed by hyperexcitability, delirium, and tremors, terminating in generalized seizures, often followed by respiratory arrest and death. Overdoses occur in three common situations: the user who increases the dosage higher and higher in hopes of reaching the ultimate response and instead reaches the maximum tolerable dose; the "stuffer" who, in an attempt to avoid arrest, ingests large quantities of drug; and the "bodypacker" who attempts to smuggle drugs into the country by swallowing numerous drug-filled condoms or other containers.

Distinguishing intoxication with cocaine from other intoxications or psychiatric disease may at first be difficult, but, because of the short half-life of cocaine, the symptoms tend to decrease quickly. The psychotic reaction with hallucinations and violent behavior resembles a PCP intoxication, delirium tremens, and the "toxidrome"* from other sympathomimetics such as amphetamines ("speed") and phenylpropanolamine (found in diet pills).

Treatment in the overdose situation is primarily supportive. Strict attention to the ABCs is the initial goal. In the situation of the "stuffer," gastrointestinal decontamination is warranted, since the drug is usually hastily and inadequately packaged in the panic of being arrested. The "body packer" on the other hand may require surgical intervention to remove the remaining packets of drug or, if asymptomatic, may be observed in the intensive care setting until the drug-ladened packets pass. Seizures should be treated with Valium or Ativan.

Because of improved supply and market strategies, the abuse of cocaine has become commonplace. Crack, the crystalline form of the cocaine freebase, has made cocaine abuse available to even wider markets, and a rapid onset of and abatement of euphoric effects perpetuates its use. With the tremendous increase in the use and purity of cocaine available to the consumer, the number of toxic side effects and related deaths is increasing.

The onset of effects from cocaine use vary with the route of administration. Crack smoking shows the most rapid onset, within seconds of use; intravenous use within three to five minutes; and when insufflated into the nasal mucosa, peak effects are within twenty to sixty minutes.

Toxicity related to cocaine use may affect any organ system. Cardiac toxicity may present as myocardial infarction in an

---

*A clinically recognizable syndrome associated with a class of toxic ingestions.

otherwise healthy young person, and arrhythmias due to myocardial irritability may cause sudden death. Stroke syndrome, seizure, subarachnoid hemorrhage, and hyperpyrexia also may occur. Psychiatric changes include decreased rapid eye movement (REM) sleep, agitation, inability to concentrate, visual hallucinations, tactile hallucinations (cocaine bugs), delusions, and acute onset of psychosis that may outlast the intoxication. Nasal septal perforation, sexual dysfunction, and a myriad of assorted adverse effects have also been temporally related to cocaine use. Toxic effects including death have been seen with a variety of dosages, even as low as 20 mg or the equivalent of one "line," and with all routes including intranasal.

Hypertension (a common problem with overdose) has been treated with nitroprusside, phentolamine, and propranolol. Supraventricular tachycardia and ventricular tachycardia have been successfully treated with intravenous propranolol, but because of the rapid degradation of cocaine, a shorter half-life agent such as esmolol may be more beneficial. Hyperpyrexia, which is an uncommon side effect, should be managed aggressively with rapid cooling.

REFERENCES
Textbook   Rosen. Pp. 2173–2181.

Review Article   Gawin, F. H., and Ellinwood, E. H. Cocaine and other stimulants. *N. Engl. J. Med.* 1988;318:1173–1182.

Additional   McCarron, M. N., and Wood, J. D. The cocaine body packer
References   syndrome. *J.A.M.A.* 1983;220:1417–1420.

Isner, J. M., et al. Acute cardiac events temporarily related to cocaine abuse. *N. Engl. J. Med.* 1986;315:1438–1443.

Derlet, E. R., and Albertson, T. E. Emergency department presentation of cocaine intoxication. *Ann. Emerg. Med.* 1989;18: 182–186.

Hoffman, R. S., et al. Whole bowel irrigation and the cocaine body-packer: A new approach to a common problem. *Am. J. Emerg. Med.* 1990;8:523–527.

Case 23 Nosebleed

A 64-year-old man was brought to the emergency department because of a nosebleed. His nose had been bleeding on and off for two days. He had placed some cotton in the left nostril for a few hours the day before his ED visit but then removed it. He was on no drugs, denied alcoholism, and had no known hypertension. There was no trauma to the nose, and family members who brought in the patient reported that he had been complaining of feeling tired that day.

The patient was placed on a bed with his head elevated. His blood pressure was 124/76 and pulse 70. He had a slow ooze of blood from his left nostril and sat clutching a blood-soaked terry-cloth towel. When he was stood up, he became dizzy and his blood pressure dropped to 70 systolic. No diastolic pressure was recorded. His pulse did not speed up noticeably on standing briefly. The inside of his left nostril was sprayed liberally with 4% cocaine, and then 4% cocaine was applied by cotton (twisted on a wire) into the nose. The left nostril was suctioned, but no precise bleeding point could be identified. A nasal pack with petroleum jelly—impregnated gauze was placed, and the bleeding stopped. An intravenous infusion of normal saline solution was given through a large intracatheter in the patient's left arm; 2000 ml was given over one hour. Blood was sent for type and crossmatch (4 units were set up). The patient was admitted to the hospital for observation overnight.

How much blood is usually lost by epistaxis?

If bleeding stops after spraying phenylephrine (a vasoconstrictor) in the nose, should you pack the nose?

How long should the pack be left in place?

DISCUSSION   Epistaxis is probably the most common ear-nose-throat emergency. Although nonphysicians usually overestimate blood loss,
exsanguination via epistaxis can occur, and the physician
should seek evidence of hypovolemia. Initial vital signs may be
normal, but the physician should look for a drop in blood pressure or elevation of pulse rate when the patient sits or stands
from a lying position. The patient should immediately resume
the supine position if light-headedness occurs. Intravenous access should be obtained if hypovolemia is present and fluid
resuscitation with normal saline or lactated Ringer's begun prior
to further evaluation of the bleeding source.

Epistaxis may be influenced by local and systemic factors.
Local factors include nasal trauma (fractures, nose picking),
ulcers from nasal dryness, nasopharyngeal tumors, foreign bodies, and even hereditary hemorrhagic telangiectasia (Osler-We-
ber-Rendu disease). Systemic factors include hypertension, ar-
teriosclerosis, blood dyscrasias, and coagulation disorders,
including nonsteroidal anti-inflammatory drug use and anticoagulant therapy. A thorough history and physical examination should provide clues to the diagnosis. In young persons
with no other medical problems, a spun hematocrit may be the
only test required, but full laboratory evaluation including platelet count, clotting studies (PT, PTT), hematocrit, and blood typing and crossmatch should be considered.

Examination is best done with the patient in the sitting position and with the head tilted forward to reduce swallowing and
potential aspiration of blood. The nasal septum, roof, and lateral walls should be inspected for a source of bleeding using a
nasal speculum, headlamp, and suction. Anterior epistaxis most
frequently originates from Kiesselbach's plexus on the anteroin-
ferior septum because of its rich vascularity and propensity for
local trauma. Posterior epistaxis tends to cause bleeding into the
nasopharynx.

You will often be successful at stopping anterior epistaxis
simply by pinching the nose continuously for fifteen to twenty
minutes. If bleeding continues, a topical vasoconstrictor such as
phenylephrine and a topical anesthetic such as 4% lidocaine
should be sprayed or applied topically to the nasal mucosa with
a cotton pledget. Topical cocaine solutions provide both vasoconstriction and anesthesia but can cause toxic effects such as
seizures or hypertension if too much is given. Large intranasal
clots should be removed and bleeding sites can then be cau-
terized with silver nitrate, or have hemostatic materials (Sur-
gicel, Gelfoam) applied to them. If the bleeding is not controlled

at that point, anterior packing is performed using a hemostatic nasal balloon or petrolatum gauze. Gauze packing is inserted using bayonet forceps. Half-inch gauze strips are layered into the nostril beginning at the nasal floor until it is fully packed. Ampicillin or cephalosporin should be started to prevent sinusitis from obstruction of sinus drainage. The patient with a unilateral anterior pack is usually sent home and asked to return for pack removal in forty-eight to seventy-two hours. Patients with multiple bleeding sites who require bilateral anterior packs deserve admission and observation.

Posterior epistaxis persists after anterior nasal packing and usually requires otolaryngologic consultation. Patients with posterior nasal packing, especially if elderly, require admission because of the risk of airway compromise and ventilatory impairment.

REFERENCES
Textbook   Rosen. Pp. 410–417.

Review   Nose Bleed. In D. D. DeWeese, W. H. Saunders (eds.), *Textbook of Otolaryngology*, 6th edition. St. Louis, Mosby, 1982. Pp. 189–200.

Additional   Walike, J. W., and Chinn, J. Evaluation and treatment of acute
Reference   bleeding from the head and neck. *Otolaryngol. Clin. North Am.* 1979;12:455–464.

Case 24 "Lockjaw"

A 34-year-old woman walked into the emergency department accompanied by her aunt. The patient was obviously very frightened, and tears were running down her face, but she spoke with very little movement of her mouth and claimed that she had "lockjaw." The aunt furnished the following information: the patient had been well until one week earlier, when she had had some cramping low abdominal pain and nausea. She had seen her physician, who had given her some yellow capsules. The pain and nausea had lessened, but for the past two days she had had trouble using her mouth, and today it had "locked on her." She recalled no trauma or puncture wounds and denied any experimental use of drugs, "pill popping," or "shooting up" of drugs. The yellow pills were unavailable.

On examination the vital signs were observed as follows: temperature 37.0°C, pulse 100, blood pressure 140/85, respiration 18. The patient's chest and heart were normal, and deep tendon reflexes were normal. Her gait was unremarkable, and muscle tone seemed normal. Her jaw was tightly clenched, but on coaxing she could open it for examination. No pharyngeal, ear, or neck pathology could be found.

One of the examining physicians at first thought the patient had a peritonsillar abscess or, failing that, a hysterical conversion reaction. To add to the confusion, the woman's aunt was loudly chanting prayers for her relief. Fortunately, an alert nurse correctly diagnosed the problem. The patient was given an intravenous injection and immediately remarked that she felt better. Within five minutes the jaw tightness was entirely gone. The patient left for home within thirty minutes of her arrival in the ED.

What was the matter with this woman?

What was in the yellow capsules?

What drug was given to her in the ED?

DISCUSSION   The patient exemplifies an acute onset of an extrapyramidal movement disorder, an acute dystonic reaction. This is usually due to phenothiazines and is essentially unrelated to the dose, being an idiosyncratic reaction. The differential diagnosis must include (1) tetanus, (2) a seizure disorder, and (3) hysteria. Indeed, the unsophisticated physician usually picks hysteria as an explanation for phenothiazine reactions, and at one time almost all extrapyramidal diseases were thought to be hysterical since the movements are exacerbated by anxiety, improved by tranquillity, and *partially* under the patient's control.

These movement disorders can present as dystonias such as torticollis, oculogyric crisis (the patient may complain that she cannot get her eyes off the ceiling), or total body writhing. The patient may have spasmodic movements with leg-jerking, head-bobbing, or choreiform total body hyperactivity. Localized muscle tone increases may vary from this patient's sense of jaw tightness or tongue protrusion to opisthotonos and extensor rigidity throughout the body.

Probably any phenothiazine can lead to movement disorders, although Haldol does so more commonly than most. Several effective therapies are available. The offending drug must be stopped. If the movement disorder is of recent onset, diphenhydramine (Benadryl) given orally or intravenously will rapidly reduce symptoms. We usually give 50 mg intravenously to produce a dramatic improvement that is very reassuring to the patient. Then we continue the patient on 25 to 50 mg orally bid for two or three days. This was the therapy used on the patient described.

REFERENCES
Textbook   Rosen. Pp. 1870–1871.

Review Article Lee, A. Treatment of drug induced dystonic reaction. *JACEP* 1979;8:453–457.

Additional   Denetropoullos, S., and Schauben, J. L. Acute dystonic reac-
References   tion from "street Valium". *J. Emerg. Med.* 1987;5:293–297.

Bailie, G. R. et al. Unusual treatment response of a dystonia to diphenhydramine. *Ann. Emerg. Med.* 1987;16:705–708.

Case 25 Hyperventilation: The Anxious Divorcee

A 29-year-old woman came to the emergency department complaining of "hyperventilating." She had suffered for years from chronic anxiety and had previously had many anxiety attacks accompanied by rapid breathing and weakness. Sometimes she would have paresthesias, and she had learned to treat the attacks by breathing in a paper bag. Aside from a regular alcohol consumption of several drinks daily, she had no other known medical problems.

On the day before her ED visit, as she was driving home from the divorce court—where she had just obtained a final divorce decree—she noted the onset of rapid breathing with a sense of dyspnea and within minutes noted the onset of a pounding, rapid heartbeat in her chest. She felt weak but continued driving home. Bag breathing gave her no relief. None of her previous episodes of hyperventilation had been accompanied by palpitations. Eighteen hours later, at 4 A.M., she became worried enough about the palpitations, dyspnea, tachypnea, and weakness to call for an ambulance to bring her to the ED.

On arrival the patient was anxious and in some evident distress. She was afebrile and showed acrocyanosis with cool extremities. She had a deep rapid respiration (a rate of 35), tachycardia (cardiac rate 160 and regular), and blood pressure of 150/85. Her jugular venous pressure seemed normal. She had a clear chest, unremarkable heart sounds, and no edema. A brief neurologic exam showed no abnormality. She had no facial twitching on tapping the facial nerve just anterior to the ear (Chvostek's sign) and no carpal spasm on placing a blood pressure cuff around the upper arm and holding it at 170 mm Hg for three minutes (Trousseau's sign).

An ECG showed a regular supraventricular tachycardia that the physician present thought was paroxysmal atrial tachycardia (PAT). Carotid massage and gagging maneuvers produced no change. An intravenous route was established, and the patient was given digoxin, 0.5 mg intravenously. Neither this nor subsequent carotid massage nor a further 0.5 mg of digoxin led to any change. An arterial blood gas sample was obtained and showed a pH of 7.08, pCO_2 18, pO_2 110. The acidosis was noted and thought to be a lactic acidosis resulting from tissue hypoperfusion due to the tachycardia. Physostigmine (2 mg) was given intravenously, followed by ampules of $NaHCO_3$ (44 mEq each), with no change in her condition. Edrophonium (Tensilon) (10 mg) was given intravenously, and the patient's cardiac rate slowed from 160 to 130. This was thought to be remarkable—since PAT always converts abruptly or does not change at all—and redirected attention to her acidosis. She denied ingesting methanol, antifreeze, or aspirin. A urinalysis was done and showed glucose (4+) and a large amount of acetone. She was admitted to the ward with the diagnosis of diabetic ketoacidosis in a previously undiagnosed diabetic. Later she recalled that her mother had adult-onset diabetes.

What possibilities did the arterial blood gas levels reveal?

Is there any danger in bicarbonate therapy of the acidosis?

What is the danger of digitalis in an acidotic patient?

DISCUSSION   Hyperventilation is too often identified as a psychological problem, whereas it frequently is caused by serious lung disease or a
metabolic acidosis. The differential diagnosis of hyperventilation includes primary lung disorders such as asthma, congestive
heart failure, pulmonary embolism (a very frequently missed
diagnosis), and metabolic disorders. The presence of hyperventilation *with other abnormal vital signs* should suggest one of
these disorders as the primary cause. Psychological hyperventilation is a diagnosis of exclusion made after organic causes
have been ruled out.

A normal pCO_2 at sea level is about 40 mm Hg. A slight
hyperventilation produces a slight decrease of the pCO_2 to
about 37 mm Hg. This patient showed a marked decrease of
the pCO_2, thus might have been expected to show an alkalosis.
Since the patient was not only not alkalotic but was severely
acidotic, she had a metabolic acidosis.

Metabolic acidosis has four main causes. One is diabetic ketoacidosis, and the cardinal error in this case seemed to be ne-
glecting to do a urinalysis when presented with a hyperventilating patient. If a urine specimen had been examined, the
diagnosis would have been apparent before costly time was
wasted and potentially dangerous maneuvers undertaken. Other causes of metabolic acidosis are exogenous poisons (especially methanol and salicylate), renal disease with uremia or
renal tubular acidosis, and lactic acidosis (usually with gross
tissue hypoxia and often due to shock).

Treatment of severe metabolic acidosis with $NaHCO_3$ is reasonable and can lessen the risk of fatal cardiac arrhythmias;
however, the HCO_3 is denied easy access to the cerebrospinal
fluid (CSF), and the brief increase of pCO_2 by the reaction

$$H^+ + HCO_3^- \rightleftarrows H_2CO_3 \rightleftarrows H_2O + CO_2$$

will allow for an increased CSF pCO_2 and a paradoxical increase in H^+ concentration in the CSF—thus a decrease in
CSF pH. This may produce coma or seizures, so bicarbonate
therapy should be given sparingly and only if the pH is less than
7.1.

Digitalis is a dangerous drug. It can produce serious arrhythmias, especially if given in a setting of hypoxia or acidosis.
Although useful in treating a patient with PAT, use of digitalis in
a setting of sinus tachycardia and acidosis can be hazardous
and not helpful. Verapamil is the drug of choice in a hemodynamically stable patient. (Electrical countershock is the initial

therapy of choice in the unstable patient.) Physostigmine and Tensilon have no place in the modern treatment of PAT.

REFERENCES
Textbook   Tintinalli. Pp. 490–495.

Review Article   Krane, E. J. Diabetic ketoacidosis: Biochemistry, physiology, treatment, and prevention. *Pediatr. Clin. North Am.* 1987; 34:935–960.

Additional   Foster, D. W., and McGarry, J. E. The metabolic derangement
Reference   and treatment of diabetic ketoacidosis. *N. Engl. J. Med.* 1983; 309:159–169.

Case 26 Rescued from a Fire

A 53-year-old woman was pulled out of a burning apartment by fire fighters. She was not unconscious after the rescue but had no memory of what had caused the fire. She had smoked cigarettes almost for forty years and admitted to having a chronic smoker's cough. She complained of pain in her arms and upper chest where her clothing was burned, but she denied any shortness of breath and said that, except for the pain, she felt completely well.

Her initial vital signs were blood pressure 156/84, pulse 96, and respirations 24. She had second-degree burns over her shoulders, upper chest, and anterior upper arms with surrounding first-degree burns down to the elbows. Her trauma exam was otherwise unremarkable, and the remainder of the physical exam showed only somewhat coarsened breath sounds with an increased expiratory phase.

The blisters were debrided and treated with silver sulfadiazine cream and sterile dressings. She was given 2000 ml of lactated Ringer's solution over a three-hour period. The emergency department became quite busy and she was mostly ignored for the next five hours, during which time another 1000 ml of intravenous fluid slipped in.

At this time the resident responsible for her care decided that she was well enough to go home. The attending physician, having just arrived on duty, spoke to the patient who volunteered that she was a bit short of breath. Her respiratory rate was 28 per minute and wheezes were audible. Despite the protestations of the resident, the patient was admitted to the surgical intensive care unit for observation. Forty minutes after arrival in the intensive care unit, the patient began to cough up frothy fluid and was diagnosed as having pulmonary edema. She was treated with diuretics and oxygen and was allowed to rest in a semiseated position. She was discharged eight days later to be followed in the burn clinic for outpatient treatment of her burns.

What are the priorities in burn management?

What burns can be treated in an outpatient setting?

What are the respiratory complications of burns, and how should they be treated?

DISCUSSION   The state of the airway is our first concern in a burn case, just as it is in other major emergencies. If there is any clinical evidence of an airway burn, the patient should either be intubated prophylactically or examined with direct laryngoscopy to assess damage to the airway. The signs of significant airway burns include severe burns in or around the mouth, singed nasal hairs, hoarseness or stridor, dyspnea, and expectoration of carbonaceous sputum. Burns from fires in a confined area and high-pressure steam burns to the face are likely to be associated with airway compromise.

The next priority is establishing intravenous access, usually with two large-bore intravenous lines. In most serious burns, large amounts of fluid are lost, and it is easy to get behind in the patient's fluid replacement. An estimate of the fluid requirements can be obtained by formula, but ongoing fluid management must be gauged by the urine output and the level of the central venous pressure assessed clinically or measured directly.

Burns in enclosed areas also produce smoke inhalation injury. A variety of direct pulmonary irritants can produce noncardiac pulmonary edema. Carboxyhemoglobin levels should be obtained in anyone with altered mental status, especially if the burn occurred in a closed area, and elevated levels or signs of neurologic dysfunction should prompt consideration for emergency use of a hyperbaric chamber. Cyanide is formed whenever plastic burns and should be suspected in any patient with an altered level of consciousness and a severe metabolic acidosis. Treatment is with a commercially available cyanide treatment kit.

The burn should be covered with a sterile dry "burn sheet." Ice is not necessary and will actually risk increasing the depth of the burn. The extent of a burn is usually estimated by a chart using the rule of nines. In small children or persons with irregular burns, the body surface area involved can be estimated by using the patient's hand as guide. One side of a person's hand is approximately 1% of their body surface area. If an extremity burn is circumferential, neurovascular compromise can result. Circumferential chest burns can result in respiratory embarrassment due to restriction of ventilation. In either of these cases, escharotomy may be needed on an urgent basis to allow expansion of the tissues.

Electrical burns and inhalation injuries should be admitted to the hospital, as should all patients with burns over 20% of the body surface area; patients with serious burns of the hands, feet, or genitalia; and patients with accompanying injuries or serious medical conditions.

First-degree burns such as sunburn are superficial and cause only erythema; second-degree burns are into the dermis and cause blistering; third-degree burns go through the dermis and are characterized by insensate (numb) areas, which are blackened or covered with a hard, leatherlike eschar.

Small burns can be treated on an outpatient basis. First-degree and superficial second-degree burns can be treated with cool water followed by the application of antibacterial ointment or cream. Blisters can be left intact but should be peeled away if they have burst. The skin can then be treated with an antibacterial such as silver sulfadiazine and kept covered. Narcotic analgesics should be considered for pain relief. Third-degree burns and electrical burns, which are typically deeper and more extensive than they appear on the surface, usually require subspecialty consultation for definitive care.

REFERENCES

Textbook Rosen. Pp. 573–607.

Review Articles Warden, G. D. Outpatient care of thermal injuries. *Surg. Clin. North Am.* 1987;67:147–157.

Mosley, S. Inhalation injuries: A review of the literature. *Heart and Lung* 1988;17:3–9.

Additional References Harvey, J. S., et al. Emergent burn care. *South. Med. J.* 1984;77:204–214.

Jones, J., McCullen, M. J., and Dougherty, J. Toxic smoke inhalation. *Am. J. Emerg. Med.* 1987;5:317–321.

Case 27 The Morning After a Snowstorm

The morning after a snowstorm, a family of four presented to the emergency department with the following complaints: The father, a 30-year-old medical researcher, had headaches and passed out once for a few minutes. He also complained of abdominal pain and nausea and had vomited several times. His wife was very drowsy and had a severe headache. The children seemed fine. They lived in a rural area, and when their electricity went out in the storm, they switched on a small gasoline-powered generator.

The father's blood pressure was 150/90, his pulse 100, and respirations 24. Otherwise, he appeared entirely normal. His wife also had a completely normal examination. Their carboxyhemoglobin levels were 30% and 22%, respectively. These figures were extrapolated backward to the time of their exposure, estimating maximum exposure levels of 40% and 30%. They were both treated with 100% oxygen by face masks for four hours. Repeat carboxyhemoglobin levels were then 4% and 1%. They refused permission for blood gases to be drawn on the children since the examination of the children was completely normal.

Twenty-four hours later the wife called up and said that her husband was behaving violently and seemed to have lost his memory. The husband corroborated these symptoms and was very upset about them. The wife and children were acting normally. He was immediately referred to the nearest hyperbaric chamber (100 miles away) where he was given two "dives" to 3 atmospheres at 100% oxygen. This completely reversed his symptoms although he stated that it still took him a second or two more than usual to recognize persons he knew and to remember their names.

How would you recognize carbon monoxide poisoning?

What is the significance of elevated carboxyhemoglobin levels?

When is hyperbaric oxygen treatment required for carbon monoxide poisoning?

DISCUSSION   Carbon monoxide is colorless, odorless, and tasteless, and poisoning by it has few pathognomonic symptoms or signs. Patients with mild intoxication complain of nonspecific symptoms such as headache, nausea, vomiting, and dizziness. It may be misconstrued as a flu-like illness by physicians since several members of the same family often present to the ED simultaneously.

A thorough environmental history may facilitate the diagnosis. Victims found in automobiles, residing in rooms heated by oil-powered furnaces, or using charcoal-powered hibachis should be suspect.

Carbon monoxide binds to hemoglobin with an affinity 250 times greater than oxygen. The remaining oxygen molecules bind to hemoglobin more tightly, shifting the oxyhemoglobin dissociation curve to the left. The net result is tissue hypoxia and lactic acidemia from the body's attempt to compensate through anaerobic metabolism.

The carboxyhemoglobin level, a measure of the percentage of hemoglobin bound by carbon monoxide, can rapidly be obtained by most EDs. The level can be misleadingly low if significant time elapses between the exposure and the blood test, or if oxygen was administered. The symptoms of carbon monoxide poisoning can be roughly correlated with carboxyhemoglobin levels. Headache is the primary manifestation at levels of 15 to 30%; dizziness, nausea, and confusion occur at 30 to 40%; and coma develops at 50 to 60%. Death is likely at levels greater than 70%.

Other tests can lead one to suspect carbon monoxide poisoning. A venous blood sample may appear redder than normal due to the binding of carbon monoxide to hemoglobin. The arterial blood gas may reveal a low pH due to lactic acidosis. The arterial pO_2 should remain high since it measures the amount of oxygen dissolved in the blood and not the amount bound to hemoglobin. Oxygen saturation as reported by most labs is calculated from the measured PaO_2 and hemoglobin values and will also remain elevated since both these values are unaffected by carbon monoxide poisoning. In suspect cases, request that the lab *measure* the oxygen saturation. If the *measured* value is less than the *calculated* value, a "saturation gap" exists, giving a differential diagnosis of carbon monoxide poisoning, cyanide poisoning, or methemoglobinemia.

The management of carbon monoxide poisoning is administration of 100% oxygen by nonrebreather face mask. This reduces the half-life of carboxyhemoglobin from five hours to approximately eighty minutes.

The husband in this case developed a delayed neuropsychiatric syndrome manifested by personality alteration and memory loss. This syndrome is estimated to occur in 3 to 10% of patients and its mechanism is unknown. No clinical parameters reliably predict which patients will develop it, although those who lose consciousness and then later recover are at higher risk. The syndrome does not seem to occur in patients treated with hyperbaric oxygen.

Although indications for and the benefit of hyperbaric oxygenation remain controversial, some authorities recommend it if there has been a history of or presence of coma, neurologic findings other than a mild headache, a carboxyhemoglobin level greater than 25% at any time, symptoms persisting longer than four hours, or signs of the delayed neuropsychiatric syndrome. Why hyperbaric oxygen therapy helps patients with the delayed syndrome is unclear, since carbon monoxide itself is long gone from these patients by then.

REFERENCES
Textbook

Tintinalli. Pp. 51, 809–812.

Review Article

Olsen, K. R. Carbon monoxide poisoning: Mechanism, presentation, and controversies in management. *J. Emerg. Med.* 1984;1:233–243.

Additional References

Myers, R. A. M., Snyder, S. K., and Emhoff, T. A. Sub-acute sequelae of carbon monoxide poisoning. *Ann. Emerg. Med.* 1985;14:1163–1167.

Norkool, D. M., and Kirkpatrick, J. N. Treatment of acute carbon monoxide poisoning with hyperbaric oxygen: A review of 115 cases. *Ann. Emerg. Med.* 1985;14:1168–1171.

Kindwall, E. P. Hyperbaric treatment of carbon monoxide poisoning. *Ann. Emerg. Med.* 1985;14:1233–1234.

Grace, T. W., and Platt, F. W. Subacute carbon monoxide poisoning: Another great imitator. *J.A.M.A.* 1981;246:1698–1700.

Case **28** A "Fainter" Under a Doctor's Care

A 65-year-old man was brought to the emergency department by ambulance. He had passed out on a downtown sidewalk, and the ambulance was called by bystanders. On arrival, the patient insisted that he felt well. He claimed to be a "fainter." He had fainted over fifteen times in the last year. During these faints, which lasted no more than a few minutes, he was never incontinent and had no remarkable movements. There was no aura or warning, and he had never hurt himself in a fall. The man was visiting from another city, where he was under the care of a Veterans Administration hospital cardiologist for these faints. He was planning to return home the very next day and in fact had an appointment with his physician within a week. He denied any other symptoms and was on no medications.

The physical examination revealed nothing remarkable. Blood pressure was 140/80, pulse 80 and regular, respiratory rate 15, temperature 37.0°C and jugular venous pressure seemed within normal limits. The patient was alert, well-oriented, and had no gross neurologic defects. An ECG showed right bundle branch block (RBBB) and first-degree atrioventricular (AV) block with a PR interval of 0.26 seconds.

The patient wanted no therapy and minimized the event. He was discharged to return to the care of his physician in his home city. Twelve hours later he was brought back to the ED, having expired suddenly. He was dead on arrival, and no resuscitation was attempted.

What is the significance of coexistent RBBB and first-degree AV block?

What other ECG abnormalities might have the same ominous portent?

What might best have been done for the patient when he came to the ED?

DISCUSSION   Syncope, a transient loss of consciousness, in most cases lasts
less than five minutes and is caused by three basic mechanisms:
decrease in delivery of oxygen or glucose to the brain or by
seizure activity. Cardiac causes account for less than 10% of
syncope but have a high degree of lethality (30% in one year).

This patient's history is classic for Stokes-Adams attacks: loss
of consciousness that follows the development of complete
heart block with attendant ventricular fibrillation, ventricular tachycardia, bradyarrhythmia, or asystole. The arrhythmia may
be intermittent, and the patient may die during an attack, as
probably happened in this case.

Not all cardiac causes of syncope are signaled by the ECG;
however, some ECG signs are important as probable progenitors
of complete heart block and consequently the liability of sudden
death. These are RBBB with left axis deviation of the un-
blocked early QRS forces, Mobitz type-II block (complete sudden failure of a beat to conduct), alternating RBBB and left
bundle branch block (LBBB), LBBB masquerading as RBBB, and
some instances of either RBBB or LBBB with first-degree AV
block. These ECG patterns reflect bilateral bundle branch disease. It may be a small step from such bilateral disease to complete heart block, and the history of syncope bridges this gap.

In rare instances the ECG will make the diagnosis of a myocardial infarction that was silent except for the syncope. Occasionally myocardial defects or valvular lesions associated with
loss of consciousness, such as aortic stenosis, may be found
through patient history, physical examination, or ECG.

With a resting ECG abnormality suggestive of periods of severe AV block and with a history of many faints, this patient
should have been admitted to the hospital and evaluated by
clinical examination, serial ECGs, Holter or prolonged ECG
monitoring, and perhaps sophisticated electrophysiologic studies of his conducting system.

Permanent pacing is indicated in intermittent or fixed asymptomatic AV (His bundle) and trifascicular block, symptomatic
block at any site, and symptomatic bradyarrhythmic sinus node
dysfunction.

One probably should assume that any fainter might die with
the next faint. A pacemaker could be counted on to take over if
the patient's own conduction system failed. The fact that he had
not died with previous faints does not make further episodes of
AV block less dangerous. The actual mechanism of death in this
patient was not determined, but it seems most likely to have
been a blockage of AV conduction.

Syncope is a common presenting problem in most EDs. Most patients have no suggestions of a seizure in their histories, and few have helpful ECGs. Perhaps more patients should be admitted to hospitals for monitoring purposes even with normal ECGs.

REFERENCES

Textbook   Rosen. Pp. 1282–1284, 1793–1798.

Review Article   Sobel, B. E., and Roberts, R. Hypotension and Syncope. In E. Braunwald (ed.), *Heart Disease: A Textbook of Cardiovascular Medicine.* Philadelphia, Saunders, 1988. Pp. 7–8, 884–894.

Additional   Moss, A. J., and Davis, R. J. Brady-Tachy syndrome. *Prog. Car-*
References   *diovasc. Dis.* 1974;16:439–454.

Falk, R. H., Zoll, P. M., and Zoll, R. H. Safety and efficacy of noninvasive cardiac pacing: A preliminary report *N. Engl. J. Med.* 1983;309:1166–1180.

Martin, G. J., et al. Prospective evaluation of syncope. *Ann. Emerg. Med.* 1984;13:499–504.

Zoll, P. M. Resuscitation of the heart in ventricular stand still by external electrical stimulation. *N. Engl. J. Med.* 1952;248:768–771.

Case 29 "I Think I Have Pneumonia"

A 30-year-old man arrived at the emergency department stating, "I think I have pneumonia." Four days prior, after an eight-hour drive to another state, he noted sharp right-sided chest pain worse on deep inspiration. He was somewhat short of breath and had a nonproductive cough. There was no fever, no hemoptysis, and he denied any history of trauma. His past medical history was unremarkable, but he did smoke a pack of cigarettes daily. While still away from home, he presented himself to the local ED with these complaints. His workup there revealed a right basilar infiltrate that "did not look like a pneumonia" according to the physician on duty. On returning home, he received a call from the hospital stating that the radiologist had reviewed his chest film and thought that it was consistent with pneumonia. They suggested that he go to the closest ED for treatment. His symptoms had persisted unchanged despite treatment with ibuprofen. Vital signs at our hospital revealed a pulse of 120, blood pressure 120/80, respiratory rate 28, and an oral temperature of 100.2°F. Physical exam was unremarkable except for decreased breath sounds at the right base and the absence of obvious respiratory distress. Repeat chest x-ray revealed elevation of the right hemidiaphragm, right basilar atelectasis, and a small right-sided pleural effusion. His arterial blood gas results were pH 7.50, pCO_2 30, and pO_2 70 on room air. Because of the possibility of a pulmonary embolus, a lung scan was performed that revealed a matched ventilation-perfusion defect at the right base. It was interpreted as an indeterminate-probability lung scan.

What is the most common clinical sign or symptom of pulmonary embolism?

Is an arterial blood gas helpful in ruling in or out the diagnosis of anxiety with "hyperventilation syndrome"?

DISCUSSION   The diagnostic problem here is largely distinguishing between a pulmonary embolism with infarction and a pneumonia with effusion. If embolism is the correct diagnosis, the danger is that another, larger embolus may be forthcoming and may prove fatal. The problem is usually not *this* embolus but the next one.

The triad of chest pain (usually pleuritic), shortness of breath, and hemoptysis is usually not present, although shortness of breath is the single most common symptom and is present in 84% of patients with pulmonary emboli. Historical factors suggesting the presence of pulmonary embolus are a period of prolonged immobilization, malignancy, recent surgery, prior history of phlebitis, or birth control pill use, although often none of these are present. This patient had no marked immobilization but had been on a long car trip. The type of pain does not distinguish between a pulmonary embolism and pneumonia. Pneumonia may lead to a productive cough, but may present with a dry cough. Hemoptysis can occur with pneumonia or pulmonary embolism with infarction but only occurs in 30% of patients with embolism. The most common ECG finding in either syndrome is sinus tachycardia, and the pulmonary embolism "classic" finding of an S wave in lead I, Q in III, and inverted T in III ($S_1Q_3T_3$) is rarely seen. The chest x-ray in pulmonary embolism will usually be abnormal. It may show a characteristic lack of vascular markings (Westermark's sign) or a dome-shaped opacity that is concave toward the hilum (Hampton's hump). Usually it just shows nonspecific abnormalities such as a small effusion, infiltrate, or atelectasis.

An arterial blood gas analysis may show hypoxemia with normal or low pCO_2 in either disease state. A normal arterial blood sample might be found at this time, four days into his history. A lung scan can be done and is helpful if it shows filling defects in areas normal on the chest x-ray. It will probably show the defect seen on the x-ray in either disorder. If the scan shows other defects, pulmonary emboli are probable.

The absence of peripheral venous obstruction signs or symptoms is in no way a significant argument against the diagnosis of pulmonary embolism and infarction. Venous findings are present in less than half the cases of documented pulmonary emboli. The most helpful cardiac finding arguing for pulmonary embolism is a loud second component of the second heart sound in the pulmonic area.

The major therapeutic dilemma is whether or not to give the patient an anticoagulant. To make this decision one may need a pulmonary angiogram. Probably the best approach in an equivocal case would be to admit the patient to the hospital for angiography and possibly heparinization. All too often such a patient has less diagnostic procedures done with equivocal results, is sent home on antibiotics, and suffers a recurrence of pulmonary embolism. Pulmonary angiography in this patient showed an occlusion of the right lower lobe pulmonary artery, and heparin anticoagulation was begun.

In the hyperventilation syndrome, there is no alveolar-arterial (a-A) oxygen gradient. Thus hyperventilation results in a higher than normal pO_2 and a low pCO_2. The a-A gradient at sea level can be estimated by the formula $145 - (pO_2 + pCO_2)$. This should be less than 10 to 20 mm Hg in normal persons but can be elevated in smokers and persons with other lung diseases.

REFERENCES
Textbook   Tintinalli. Pp. 218–221.

Review Article   Goldhaber, S. Z., and Braunwald, E. Pulmonary Embolism. In E. Braunwald (ed.), *Heart Disease: A Textbook of Cardiovascular Medicine.* Philadelphia, Saunders, 1988. Pp. 1577–1596.

Additional   Valenzuela, T. D. Pulmonary embolism. *Ann. Emerg. Med.*
References   1988;17:209–213.

West, J. W. Pulmonary embolism. *Med. Clin. North Am.* 1986;70:877–894.

Fulkervson, W. et al. Diagnosis of pulmonary embolism. *Arch. Intern. Med.* 1986;146:961–967.

PIOPED investigators. Value of the ventilation/perfusion scan in acute pulmonary embolism. *JAMA* 1990;263:2753–2795.

Case 30 Headaches

A 30-year-old man, a psychologist, came to the emergency department complaining of severe left-sided throbbing headaches over the preceding two weeks. His headaches involved the left face from brow to maxilla and centered about the left eye. During headaches that lasted for several hours, he often vomited, and this seemed to relieve the pain somewhat. He had no family history of headache, no juvenile carsickness or frequent nausea, and recalled no head trauma. He noted that one of his more severe episodes had followed an alcoholic drink, but usually he did not drink or smoke. Although one headache had awakened him, the rest had been during the daytime hours. About three years earlier he had suffered several similar headaches over a two-month period. He was on no drugs except aspirin, which gave him little relief.

On physical examination he appeared to be a normal man in no apparent distress. Vital signs were normal: temperature 37.0°C and blood pressure 130/80. His pain was now gone, and his conjunctivae were normal, although he thought the left eye was sometimes bloodshot with the pain. There were no audible bruits over the skull and no tenderness over the sinuses, and fundi and tympanic membranes were normal. His neck was supple, and the patient appeared entirely normal on a careful neurologic exam and a brief general physical exam.

What should be examined when a patient complains of headache?

What sort of headache syndromes are most common in the ED?

When does a patient deserve a spinal tap?

What is the diagnosis in this case?

DISCUSSION   The patient information needed to evaluate a case of headache
includes the following: Where is the headache? Is it unilateral or
bilateral? Does it pound with the pulse, or is it a steady headache? (It is important to avoid using the word "only" in discuss-
ing this matter with the patient, as in "Is your headache pounding or *only* steady?") Does the patient have a fever or chills?
Has he been suffering from upper respiratory symptoms such
as runny nose, stuffy head, earache, ringing in ears, sore throat,
or hoarseness? Was there any previous head trauma? Has he
been having blurred or double vision, nausea, or vomiting? Has
he had high blood pressure in the past? What drugs is he taking
and what is he allergic to? Does coughing or sneezing exacer-
bate the headache? Is there photophobia? How does he try to
relieve the pain? Are there any warnings before the headache?
Have his previous headaches ever been this severe? Is this the
worst headache of his life?

The important physical findings to elicit in any case of headache include the vital signs, a thorough head and neck exam,
and a neurological exam. Be sure to check for tenderness of the
skull and the maxillary and frontal sinuses. The frontal sinuses
must be felt from under the supraorbital ridge as opposed to
the maxillary sinuses, which can be palpated directly. Check the
equality of the pupils and their response to light. Evaluate the
presence of nystagmus. Check flexibility of the neck with the
patient attempting to put his ears on his shoulders and to flex
his chin on his chest. Observe his gait and look for any lateralizing neurological signs. Examine the optic fundi for papilledema
or hemorrhages.

Headache syndromes that present in the ED include the following:

1. Febrile headaches—usually bilateral and present with a fever
   of at least 38.4°C. This headache may be steady but is often
   pounding. Of course, the source of the fever must be found,
   and this may turn out to be as simple as a urinary tract
   infection, respiratory tract infection, or viral syndrome.
2. Muscular headache—usually bilateral and mainly in the back
   of the head. It is steady and worse in the evening. It may last
   for days. It is the most common headache syndrome seen
   and usually responds to salicylates or other mild pain medications, such as Darvon, and to adjunctive measures such as
   rest, relaxation, or heat to the back of the neck.
3. Vascular headaches—usually classified as (a) atypical or
   common migraine or (b) typical or uncommon migraine.

The point of this is that the vascular headache usually seen does not have all the features of classic migraine. The classic migraine headache is a unilateral, pounding headache with visual changes, nausea, and vomiting; it lasts for hours, and there is a strong family history of headaches. The more common varieties often lack some of these features and may have no prodrome. In addition, a vascular headache often eventually develops into a muscular headache. A number of drugs are being used with some success to treat these headaches prophylactically. Aspirin, propranolol, tricyclic antidepressants, and other drugs all have a role. Once the headache has progressed, the best treatment used to be strong analgesics, especially narcotics. A new, alternative treatment is a dose of prochlorperazine (Compazine) or chlorpromazine (Thorazine) given slowly intravenously. It is often surprisingly effective, and avoids the use of narcotics.

4. Sinus headaches—rare. Many patients who come in complaining of sinus headaches are actually complaining of other sorts of headaches. If the patient indeed has a fever and is tender over the sinuses, a set of sinus films should be obtained. In adults, sinusitis is usually caused by streptococcal infections or viral infections. *Haemophilus influenzae* is a common pathogen in children and adolescents and is becoming more common in adults. Treatment should, of course, include antibiotics if the physician suspects bacterial sinusitis. Usually the microbial etiology will be unclear and a broad-spectrum antibiotic such as amoxicillin or cefaclor is the antibiotic of choice. Important adjuncts in treatment are analgesics and decongestants.

5. Hypertension headache—generally in the back of the head and often worse in the morning. The diastolic blood pressure should be at least 110 mm Hg to make this diagnosis. The problem is increased by the fact that many people get a temporary elevation of the diastolic blood pressure with pain anywhere, including headache. Headache alone is not a sign of hypertensive emergency, although signs of central nervous system, renal, or cardiac decompensation should be looked for.

6. Post head-trauma headache—often involves the entire head. Patients who have been hit on the head (especially if they have suffered concussion) may have a syndrome consisting of headache, light-headedness, and malaise that can last for weeks. The patient's affect may be depressed,

and he may find himself "neurotic" and unable to do his usual work. As long as the patient is continuing to improve the most important part of the therapy is reassurance. The patient should be told that this syndrome often occurs following head trauma and that it always goes away.

7. Although eye problems are often suggested, they are very rare as a cause of headache. Nevertheless, glaucoma should be kept in mind.

8. Dental problems also can cause headaches in rare instances, but one should consider trigeminal neuralgia or temporal mandibular joint arthritis.

Any headache patient who has remarkable physical findings and who does not seem to fit clearly in any of the above categories may have more serious organic brain disease. The physical examination recommended here for headache workup is actually quite brief and can be done in about four minutes. Headache patients may need further workup for disorders such as brain tumor and other intracranial pathology. Patients making *repeated* visits for severe headache without a clear diagnosis usually deserve to have at least one computed tomography scan and a spinal tap. The adage "When you think of it, do it" holds most of the time for a spinal tap. A patient who says that his present headache is *the worst he has ever had* probably deserves a tap to rule out meningitis or a subarachnoid hemorrhage. Another possibility, particularly in the era of acquired immunodeficiency syndrome, is that the headache may be due to chronic meningitis or a mass lesion such as a brain abscess. A lumbar puncture (LP) in these patients can cause herniation and death. Consequently a very close look for papilledema, and preferably a computed tomography scan, is essential before the LP in these cases.

In this case the patient probably had a vascular headache known as cluster migraine or Horton's histamine cephalalgia. Therapy with Cafergot (ergotamine plus caffeine) aborted many of his subsequent headaches, but he still eventually needed therapy with methysergide (Sansert).

REFERENCES

Textbook　　　　Rosen. Pp. 279–293.

Review Article　　Diamond, S., and Freidman, A. *Headache. Continuing Patient Management Series.* New Hyde Park, NY, Medical Exam, 1983.

Additional References　　Kunkel, R. S. Evaluating the headache patient: History and workup. *Headache* April 1979, 122–126.

Packard, R. C. What does the headache patient want? *Headache* November 1979;370–374.

Gower, D. J., et al. Contraindications to lumbar puncture as defined by computed cranial tomography. *J. Neurol. Neurosurg. Psychiatry* 1987;50:1071–1074.

Iserson, K. V. Parenteral chlorpromazine treatment of migraine. *Ann. Emerg. Med.* 1983;12:756–758.

Case 31 "DTs"

A 36-year-old man was brought to the emergency department by a concerned friend who promptly vanished. The patient claimed that he was "going into the DTs." He had been drinking heavily for about sixteen years and had been dry for no more than four months at a time during that period. His present binge had lasted three weeks. He had been drinking mainly vodka at a rate of over a fifth a day, but the past few days he had been drinking wine, and today his money had run out. His last drink had been six hours before he came to the ED. Between binges he had worked as a laborer, dishwasher, and cook. He smoked two packs of cigarettes a day and admitted to having "a smoker's cough." During the preceding few days he had been nauseated and had vomited several times, especially in the mornings. The vomiting did not follow a coughing spell, and after taking a drink ("the hair of the dog that bit him"), he felt better. Now he felt shaky, nauseated, and generally very sick. He claimed to be hallucinating when left alone: "seeing animals on the wall." He said he "needed a drink" and asked for an injection of Librium.

On physical examination the patient was tremulous and anxious and looked ill. He was wasted and unshaven. His right hand had multiple cigarette tar stains. His clothes smelled of urine and other unidentifiable odors. Vital signs included blood pressure 160/110 in the right arm when recumbent, 140/100 standing, pulse 130, respiratory rate 25, temperature 38.1°C. His venous pressure seemed normal. His eyes were bloodshot; his chest had audible bilateral coarse wheezes; his abdomen was diffusely moderately tender; and his legs and feet seemed inordinately sensitive to stroking or pressure. He would jerk his leg away when the sole of the foot was touched.

Why do alcoholics stop drinking?

Does this patient have delirium tremens?

Can alcohol withdrawal symptoms appear within six hours of the last drink?

DISCUSSION   The *binge drinker* can be dry for months but is drunk for days or weeks when he drinks. His binge is generally ended in one of three ways. He may be arrested by the police for "being drunk in a public place" or driving while under the influence of alcohol, and once in jail he will begin to suffer withdrawal symptoms. He may suffer an attack of acute gastritis, pancreatitis, or pneumonia that will render him too ill to continue to drink. Most commonly, he will run out of money. In this setting he may taper off over several days with wine or beer.

The earliest withdrawal symptoms are usually nausea and vomiting, notably the morning after a binge. These are treatable with alcohol or benzodiazepines and so represent withdrawal symptoms rather than gastritis or other intra-abdominal pathology. Then tremor, anxiety, and malaise become prominent. Many withdrawing alcoholics seem unable to define their symptoms beyond being "sick."

Fever is common, as is tachycardia, in alcohol withdrawal; however, almost all drinkers are heavy smokers and may be cross-addicted to other abused drugs such as cocaine and sedatives. The alcohol suppresses the white blood cell count (folate deficiency and direct bone marrow suppression) and the pulmonary mucociliary apparatus. The cigarette smoke is a chronic irritant, making the patient prone to bronchitis, pneumonia, and tuberculosis. Gastrointestinal bleeding is common in alcoholics due to increased incidence of peptic ulcers, Mallory-Weiss tears of the esophagus, gastritis, and esophageal varices. Such a patient should have pulse and blood pressure taken supine and upright to look for evidence of hypovolemia. He also must have a rectal examination and a stool test for occult blood.

Head trauma is common in alcoholics, and chronic or acute subdural hematomas are prevalent. Confusion and ataxia should not be accepted too quickly as due to alcohol intoxication. With head trauma and alcohol intoxication (a very common combination), we always do a serum ethanol level to confirm that the patient's confusion or obtundation is consistent with and therefore explained by a measured serum level. Intoxicated patients with an abnormal mental status should never be allowed to leave the ED unless supervised by a reliable observer.

Hallucinations—deranged and distorted sensory perceptions—are common in alcohol withdrawal. They may begin as nightmares, then go on to include hallucinations when the patient is alone in a dark room. Next there may be visual (seldom auditory) hallucinations even in well-lighted rooms. All these are generally ego-alien to the patient: He recognizes them as frightening but unreal. Only after many days are the hallucinations ego-syntonic and the patient truly lost within them. The early alcohol withdrawal syndrome may also include tonic-clonic seizures and an increase in sympathetic tone (increased blood pressure, pulse, diaphoresis, and tremors), which is promptly and dramatically treatable with intravenous benzodiazepines.

Delirium tremens (DT) is a rare syndrome in a withdrawing alcoholic who does not also have an associated illness such as pancreatitis or some major trauma (accidentally or surgically incurred). The DT patient is totally disoriented, agitated, and unable to remove himself from his hallucinations. He has a tachycardia and often a very high fever. He does *not* arrive able to tell us that he is "going into DTs." DT requires intensive care.

This patient seems to have an alcohol withdrawal syndrome with tremor, nausea and vomiting, tachycardia, and focal hallucinations. He also has chronic bronchitis. The alcohol withdrawal syndrome may develop even while the person is still drinking as long as his intake and blood alcohol level are dropping. One should not assume this patient's blood alcohol to be zero—he may have had several drinks more recently than he tells us.

REFERENCES

Textbook   Rosen. Pp. 2065–2086.

Review Article   West, L. J., et al. Alcoholism. *Ann. Intern. Med.* 1984;100:405–416.

Additional   Daghestani, A. N. Alcohol withdrawal: A comprehensive ap-
References   proach to treatment. *Postgrad. Med.* 1987;81:111–118.

                       Simon, R. P. Alcohol and seizures. *N. Engl. J. Med.* 1988;319:715–716.

Case 32 Blunt Trauma

A 74-year-old woman was brought to the emergency department after having been involved in a motor vehicle accident. The EMTs reported that she had turned into traffic and hit another car head on that had been traveling at approximately 50 mph. The patient was awake, alert, and breathing shallowly at a rate of 40. She complained of anterior chest and abdominal pain and a sore right knee. Her blood pressure was 130/65 with a pulse of 138. She was given oxygen and a large-bore intravenous line was started. An initial evaluation revealed no other signs of injuries. After the initial evaluation, she was sent for x-rays of her chest, cervical spine, and right knee. While in x-ray she suffered a cardiopulmonary arrest and could not be resuscitated.

How do you recognize that a real emergency is present?

DISCUSSION   Victims of multiple trauma may initially show little evidence of major malfunction, but the story of the accident or injury may suggest great violence and that violence should lead us to expect to find serious damage. Events associated with serious injury include gunshot and stab wounds, falls from heights greater than 15 feet, and surviving an accident in which someone else died. Motor vehicle accidents with impact at greater than 20 mph or where the vehicle deformity is greater than 20 inches are associated with a substantial risk of occupant injury. Anatomic injuries that suggest severe internal injuries include two or more proximal long-bone fractures, pelvic fractures, and multiple rib fractures.

Once the patient is in our hands, we can often identify the true emergencies by attention to the patient's chief complaint, mental status, and vital signs. True emergencies present as problems in the central nervous system, the respiratory system, or the cardiovascular system. Dysfunction in one of these often quickly progresses to dysfunction in all three.

To appraise brain function, the physician must make a careful neurologic and mental status examination, but a few simple questions will elicit indications of the more urgent problems: Does the patient respond to me? Is she awake? Does she know where she is, how far she is from home, what day it is, and about what time of the day it is? Is she responding appropriately to my presence, or is she struggling with and hostile to someone who is here to help her? If she is confused, hostile, or asleep and not easily roused to full alertness, then she may be a true emergency.

Adequate evaluation of the respiratory system requires only a few simple observations. What is the patient's respiratory rate? At least a full half minute should be counted. A rate under 12 or over 20 per minute should be considered a bright-red danger signal. All too often tachypnea is written off as "hyperventilation," and the correct diagnosis of pneumonia, metabolic acidosis, serious cardiovascular or pulmonary pathology, or subarachnoid hemorrhage is delayed. While the respiratory rate is counted, the regularity of respiration should be noted. A chaotic or cyclic respiratory pattern is cause for alarm. Volume of ventilation may be difficult to ascertain by watching the patient's chest or listening to it. It is easier to estimate the volume of air moved by placing a hand loosely over the patient's nose and mouth during respiration. Again, either a low or a high volume of ventilation is a serious sign. The patient's color should be gauged, and if she is dusky gray or blue, especially about the tongue and lips, she is in danger. Finally, the patient may complain of being short of breath, choking, or unable to get her breath.

Problems involving the cardiovascular system may be signaled by the most awesome physical signs, such as no palpable pulse, or may present with a normal, healthy-appearing patient who says that her chest discomfort has now vanished. Chest pain or discomfort is ominous because of its association with sudden death and myocardial infarction.

The pulse and blood pressure, especially if taken both supine and seated or upright, provide a wealth of information. An irregular pulse, or one with a rate under 50 or over 120, is a danger sign par excellence. A low blood pressure (systolic blood pressure of 100 plus patient's age will give a first approximation of the patient's blood pressure) or one that falls significantly when the patient stands is, of course, very dangerous. The mean blood pressure can be approximated by the diastolic blood pressure plus one-third of the pulse pressure. This mean should not fall 10 mm Hg on standing. A fall of 15 mm is probably dangerous and one of 20 surely significant. This maneuver will pick up hypovolemia, one of the most common pathologic processes seen in an ED as a true emergency.

There is no such thing as "just a little bit of shock." Shock is a serious problem. A drop in blood pressure due to bleeding indicates a loss of at least one-third of the total blood volume. By the time blood pressure drops, the patient is in severe shock. The initial sign of occult shock in the supine patient may be the presence of a metabolic acidosis (e.g., an initial arterial blood gas of pH 7.24, pO_2 90, pCO_2 38). Tachypnea and tachycardia, altered mental status (usually agitation), light-headedness, and thirst are later signs. Narcotics, of course, can add to the hypotension by vasodilation and should be used with *great* care if at all in a case such as this.

Fluid repletion must be done quickly with crystalloid, colloid, or blood. If the patient is in extremis, type O-negative or type-specific uncrossmatched blood should be infused until type-specific fully crossmatched blood is available. Large intravenous lines are needed. A central venous pressure catheter is helpful, but it should be a short tube in the internal jugular or subclavian vein, if fluid is to be infused rapidly through this route. The resistance of a tube is proportionate to the fourth power of its radius, so a large catheter with a diameter about twice that of a medium one can infuse fluids sixteen times as fast.

The evaluation of abdominal injuries in blunt trauma is a major challenge. Abdominal examination may be difficult for many reasons. Blood alone is not immediately irritating to the peritoneum, and significant internal bleeding may be initially present with only mild local tenderness. The unconscious patient may show no sign of peritoneal irritation. Additionally, patients who are intoxicated may show either increased or decreased perception of painful injury. Patients who exhibit significant abdominal tenderness, who are intoxicated and have a significantly serious mechanism of injury, or who have major alterations of their mental status should be considered for either a diagnostic peritoneal lavage or computed tomography (CT) of the abdomen.

Peritoneal lavage is performed with local anesthesia, usually inferior to the umbilicus. A small incision is carried down to the peritoneum, and a trochar is then gently poked through. A catheter is slipped over the trochar and aspirated. The presence of 5 ml or more of gross blood in the aspirate reveals major bleeding and is an indication for laparotomy. If there is no blood grossly, a liter of saline is infused into the abdomen and then drained out. The fluid is then sent for cell count and is considered positive if it contains more than 100,000 red blood cells per mm^3, 500 white blood cells per mm^3, or any bile, food particles, or fecal material. Great debate still continues in the literature regarding the role of CT and lavage in evaluating blunt abdominal trauma. Certainly CT is better at assessing the organ injury which is bleeding and much better at assessing the retroperitoneum (aorta, pancreas, kidneys, duodenum). Lavage is better at picking up hollow viscus injury and can be performed without moving the patient.

REFERENCES

Textbook   Tintinalli. Pp. 825–828.

Review   Committee on Trauma of the American College of Surgeons. *Advanced Trauma Life Support*. Chicago, American College of Surgeons, 1989.

Additional References   Cales, R. H., and Trunkey, D. D. Preventable trauma deaths. *J.A.M.A.* 1985;254:1059–1063.

Kearney, P. A. Blunt trauma to the abdomen. *Ann. Emerg. Med.* 1989;18:1322–1325.

Trunkey, D. D. Trauma. *Sci. Am.* 1983;249:28–35.

Matsubara, T. K. Computed tomography of abdomen in management of blunt abdominal trauma. *J. Trauma* 1990;30:410–414.

Case 33 Rectal Explosion

A 24-year-old man was brought to the emergency department by ambulance. He had placed a firecracker in his anus and lit it. The explosion brought him to the attention of bystanders, and he was brought in with a small amount of blood leaking from his anus. He had a past history of many psychiatric hospitalizations for schizophrenia and for "sexual deviancy." He had come to the ED previously with self-inflicted razor cuts of the scrotum. He had been in the state psychiatric hospital for two years for child molestation.

On physical examination the patient appeared well. There was a small mucosal tear of the anal canal and no further pathology on proctoscopic examination. Vital signs were normal.

How does one treat rectal injuries?

What parts of the treatment are most often overlooked?

DISCUSSION   We have removed from rectal ampullae a variety of foreign bodies, including pop bottles, razor blades, and electric vibrators. The trauma done to the rectum is often underestimated. A tear may lead to retroperitoneal abscess, which has a high mortality. Tears can be difficult to diagnose. A stool hematest is mandatory in these cases; fiberoptic sigmoidoscopy or even gastrografin enema may be required. Whenever doubt exists, we do a colostomy and drainage procedure. In this case the damage was limited to the anal canal and was trivial. Sitz baths alone were adequate therapy.

There is considerable rectal fascination in nonschizophrenics, and one ought not to jump to the diagnosis of schizophrenia in all patients who introduce foreign objects into the rectum. Evaluation of such patients must include attention to both ends. Careful proctoscopy must be done. If the foreign body cannot be removed with the examining finger(s), passage of a Foley catheter beyond the object, and inflation of the balloon will frequently help. Care must be taken not to do more damage. Removal of large foreign bodies may require insertion of a gloved hand with near-general anesthesia.

Preoccupation with the rectal lesion can cause the physician to forget to consult a psychiatrist, and this may be the most serious omission possible. Some attempt should be made by the emergency physician to determine if the aberration in behavior is of psychotic or organic origin. No single test is absolutely reliable in this setting, but a mental status exam will help. Three hallmarks of an organic process are disorientation, loss of a basic fund of knowledge (name of the president, governor, or other important person), and loss of the ability to do simple mathematical calculations. We find the ten-question, one-minute, organic brain syndrome quiz described by Pfeiffer and colleagues helpful.

This incident was triggered by the patient's failure to take his antipsychosis medications, which resulted in the reactivation of his psychosis. Returning him to his usual therapy was enough to achieve control of his psychotic behavior.

REFERENCES
Textbook   Rosen. Pp. 542–543.

Review Article   Bernner, B. E., and Simon, R. R. Anorectal emergencies. *Ann. Emerg. Med.* 1983;12:367–376.

Additional References

Baker, L. W. Rectal Injuries. In E. E. Moore, B. Eiseman, and C. W. Van Way (eds.), *Critical Decisions in Trauma*. St. Louis, Mosby, 1984. Pp. 214–217.

Pfeiffer, E. A. Short portable mental status questionnaire for the assessment of organic brain deficit in elderly patients. *J. Am. Geriatr. Soc.* 1975;23:433–441.

Case 34 Lost Lab Tests

A 39-year-old woman came to the emergency department complaining of abdominal pain and vomiting for two days following a day of rather heavy drinking. She denied any significant past ills but admitted that she would get an "acid stomach" if she drank two or more beers. On physical exam she appeared entirely normal except for slight diffuse abdominal tenderness. Blood pressure was 116/84 supine and 106/80 seated. Her pulse was 120 supine or seated. One ounce of Mylanta antacid gave her relief from pain, and a fingerstick hematocrit was 53%. A complete blood count and a set of electrolytes were sent to the lab but were lost there. After two hours the patient said she felt well and was sent home on a regimen of antacid, propoxyphene (Darvon) for pain, and fluids, with instructions to return if she remained ill.

Four days later she returned in severe distress. Her blood pressure was 75 systolic. Her abdomen was tense and tympanitic. Her temperature was 38.6°C. An x-ray showed free air under the diaphragm. She was hyponatremic, hypokalemic, and dehydrated. Central venous pressure was zero, and the patient was treated with high-flow intravenous fluids. After four hours she was explored. The findings included a perforated duodenal ulcer, peritonitis, and several areas of near-necrotic bowel. Despite heroic emergency measures, *Escherichia coli* and clostridial sepsis developed, and the patient died one week after exploration.

Had the ulcer perforated at the time of the patient's first ED visit?

How does one make the diagnosis of an acute abdomen requiring surgical attention?

DISCUSSION   We cannot tell retrospectively whether the patient's ulcer had
perforated on her first visit; however, pain from a distended
viscus may briefly decrease when the organ perforates. The
tachycardia suggests that she was sicker than she seemed. No
patient should be lightly discharged with an unexplained abnormal vital sign. That is often your only clue to an impending
catastrophe.

The classic features of an acute abdomen are distention, rigidity, vomiting, and pain, although all four need not be present. Distention is often written off as unimportant by patient
and physician alike by calling it "gas." Indeed gaseous distention is a sign of underlying disease. Rigidity occurs secondary to
peritoneal inflammation in patients with serious acute abdominal states such as pancreatitis, appendicitis, cholecystitis, or a
perforated viscus. It decreases with diminished alertness and
may lessen when the patient's attention is diverted. Severe abdominal pain out of proportion to physical findings in an ill-
appearing individual flags an abdominal catastrophe. Remember that acute mesenteric ischemia or ruptured abdominal aortic aneurysm may present in this manner.

Sometimes an acute abdomen can present in obscure ways,
but an alert physician with a high index of suspicion can make
the diagnosis. Especially careful assessment should be given to
the older, alcoholic, debilitated, diabetic, leukemic, and steroid-
treated patients. In these patients, the classic signs and symptoms of acute abdomen might be absent. The combination of
accurate history, physical examination, nasogastric tube placement, upright film of the abdomen or chest showing both dia-
phragms (to look for free air), and complete blood count will
help in the majority of these patients. The onset of pain before
other symptoms may be an important early hint to the presence
of an acute abdomen. Whenever there is doubt, a surgeon
should be consulted.

A positive hemeoccult test on rectal examination, or fresh
blood or "coffee grounds" on nasogastric tube placement,
would have been helpful and indicative of acute upper gastrointestinal bleed necessitating further workup. Antacid therapy is
good for symptomatic relief, but narcotic analgesics should not
be given. The analgesic given to this woman masked her abdominal pain, and the patient returned in septic shock.

REFERENCES

Textbook   Rosen. Pp. 1418–1423.

Review Article   Jordan, P. H., and Morrow C. Perforated peptic ulcer. *Surg. Clin. North Am.* 1988;68:315–329.

Additional   Norris, J. R., and Haubrich, W. S. The incidence and clinical
Reference   features of penetration in peptic ulceration. *J.A.M.A.* 1961;178:386–389.

Case 35 Diabetic in Automobile Accident

A 50-year-old man was involved in an auto accident. Seemingly unprovoked, he drove his car down a hillside into a creek. The car rolled over, and the man bounced about but stayed in the car. A police car arrived, and the officers extricated the patient. After the ambulance arrived, the EMT was able to learn from the patient that he was a diabetic. The patient was then brought to the emergency department, and the EMT told a passing nurse that he had a diabetic who had rolled his car. The nurse glanced at the patient and, deeming him "in not too bad shape," went on about her work in another room. The EMT returned to his ready room to watch television.

The patient became more confused and by the time he was seen by a physician fifteen minutes later was stuporous and could give no history. The physician arrived with a blank encounter form and an ambulance trip report that stated only "auto accident—possible injuries." The patient had no obvious signs of head injury and no focal neurologic signs but was clearly confused and stuporous. Fortunately, a youth who was in the room, waiting for his girlfriend on the next bed to be sutured, remarked that the man was a diabetic: "I heard the ambulance driver say so." A blood sugar was drawn, and 50 ml of 50% glucose solution was given intravenously. The patient became much more alert, and the blood sugar was later reported at 30 mg per dl.

What sort of information should one try to elicit from the ambulance crew, firemen, policemen, or other on-the-scene observers?

If focal neurologic signs developed in the patient, would they rule out hypoglycemia?

DISCUSSION   Patient history information is of great value to the emergency physician. All too often the patient is confused or comatose or becomes so shortly after arrival. Often no one is present who can give information about the patient. Relatives may never arrive at the ED even though they tell the ambulance attendant they are coming in, or they may leave before the physician can talk with them.

We like our EMTs to try to determine the following information and include it in the trip report for each case:

A. Trauma Patient
   1. What happened before the event? Was the patient acting strange? Did he pass out, become confused, fall, become dizzy? Did he complain of any symptoms? Was he on any drugs or other treatment? Alcohol?
   2. Description of event: If a weapon was involved, what size and sort? If a fall, how far and in what position? If an auto accident, was he seat-belted? Where was he seated? Was he thrown out? Did he hit any secondary objects? How did the accident occur? How much damage was noted on the automobile?
   3. What did he then do? Was he unconscious? Was there retrograde amnesia? Could he move his extremities? Did he complain of pain or shortness of breath? What has been the course of consciousness since the event?
   4. Other information: Whom can we contact for further information regarding the accident (a observer of the event)? Whom for background on the patient? Is he on any drugs? Is he allergic to any drugs? Is he being cared for by a physician for any chronic illness? What is the name of the physician? When did he last eat? (This must be asked should any emergent surgery be required.)
   5. How does patient now feel? What hurts (the major injury may not be the most apparent)? Trouble breathing? Confusion? Amnesia? Weakness? Dizziness?
B. Nontrauma Patient
   1. Describe major symptoms. A history taken by a neophyte tends to accept as important information the patient's own diagnosis or suggested therapy: This must be bypassed and his symptoms elicited.
   2. *Why now?* What happened to lead patient to pick this moment to seek help? Sometimes this is obvious, but if not, the question must be answered.

3. Is the patient being treated for chronic illness? Again, what is the name of the physician? What drugs is he taking, including over-the-counter medicines? (It is helpful to have the EMTs bring in any medications found in the house.) Any allergies to drugs? Who can give us more information?
4. What events occurred (and when) during ride into the ED?

The treatment of many medical emergencies can be safely begun in the field. Most EMS systems have medical control mechanisms in place that help guide the prehospital care providers. The initial care is begun under standing orders. The EMT or paramedic then contacts a base station emergency physician by radio for further orders. Remember that paramedics are trained to start intravenous lines and administer drugs, under protocol, by intravenous, endotracheal, intramuscular, subcutaneous, and oral routes. EMT training is more basic and emphasizes airway management, spinal and extremity immobilization, and rapid transport. This patient's treatment should have been started in the prehospital phase. Most EMS systems require paramedics to give intravenous glucose, naloxone (Narcan), and thiamine to any patient found with a depressed level of consciousness. Basic EMTs cannot start an intravenous line but may be able to administer glucose orally if the patient is adequately responsive.

Hypoglycemia may present in many ways. Confusion, anger, fighting, ataxia, anxiety, stupor, diaphoresis, tachycardia, or focal neurologic findings all may be present in one or another diabetic. Hypoglycemia is indeed a medical emergency and should be treated promptly. The nurse involved in this case did not realize the significance of an auto accident for a person with diabetes.

Hypoglycemia may mimic alcohol intoxication and in a busy city hospital ED is often confused with alcohol intoxication. To further confuse the issue, alcoholics with depleted hepatic glycogen stores may develop hypoglycemia even without insulin or other drug therapy. One may always draw a blood sugar and a blood alcohol, but if the diagnosis of hypoglycemia is being entertained, there is almost never any harm in giving a bolus of sugar (orally in a conscious patient or intravenously in a comatose one). We usually give 25 gm of glucose intravenously (50 cc of 50% glucose) and may repeat it once or twice. We start an intravenous infusion of 5% dextrose in water and feed the patient in the ED. The hypoglycemic action (especially with certain oral hypoglycemic drugs) may long outlast the effect of the glucose given, and the patient may lapse back into coma. Careful observation, oral sugar once awake, and instructions regarding future therapy are necessary.

Differentiating between a metabolic encephalopathy (e.g., hypoglycemia, anoxia or postanoxia, uremia, hyponatremia), a traumatic encephalopathy (e.g., postconcussion, subdural hematoma), and a toxic encephalopathy (e.g., alcohol, sedative, other drugs) can test the most adept neurologist. The patient history, as in this case, can save the day.

REFERENCES
Textbook   Tintinalli. Pp. 479–489.

Review Article   Field, J. B. Hypoglycemia. *Endocrinol. Metab. Clin. North Am.* 1989;18:27–41.

Additional   Adler, P. M. Serum glucose changes after administration of 50%
References   dextrose solution: Pre- and in-hospital calculation. *Am. J. Emerg. Med.* 1986;4:504–506.

Brodows, R. G., Williams, C., and Amatruda, J. M. Treatment of insulin reactions in diabetics. *J.A.M.A.* 1984;252:3378–3381.

Callure, A., et al. Comparison of intravenous glucagon and dextrose in treatment of severe hypoglycemia in an accident and emergency department. *Diabetes Care* 1987;10:712–715.

Case 36 Unequal Pupils

A 51-year-old man was brought to the emergency department by ambulance. He was found lying on the street, and one observer said that he may have had a seizure. On arrival in the ED, he had a pulse of 120, blood pressure 150/80, respiration rate 18, and was somnolent. He responded to deep pain by withdrawing but did not respond to voice commands. His right pupil was slightly larger than the left. He had no asymmetry of reflexes or tone, and plantar responses were flexor. "Doll's eyes" (oculocephalic responses) were not evaluated because of the possibility of a cervical spine injury. He was given 50 gm of glucose (100 ml of 50% glucose solution) by vein, and blood sugar, BUN, and electrolyte samples were drawn. There was no improvement, and shortly thereafter the patient had a generalized seizure during which he seemed to be looking to the right. A skull film showed a probable fracture, and a computed tomography (CT) scan was done but was normal. The following laboratory data were then returned: a BUN of 3 mg per 100 ml, blood sugar of 480 mg per 100 ml (unfortunately drawn after the bolus of sugar was given), and electrolytes showing a sodium concentration of 98 mEq/L, chloride 62 mEq/L, potassium 3.4 mEq/L, and bicarbonate 16 mEq/L. Treatment with 3% saline solution and potassium chloride led to arousal and then pulmonary congestion. The patient was admitted to the hospital.

What is the significance of unequal pupils after a seizure?

How low must the serum sodium be before ascribing seizures or confusion to it?

What causes hyponatremia?

DISCUSSION   Seizures may lead to unequal neurologic signs in the postictal period. Todd's paralysis or anisocoria is not unusual. The postictal findings may help define the focus of the seizures in the brain. In this case the physicians were concerned about the possibility of impending cerebral herniation due to a subdural or epidural hematoma, and an emergency CT scan was needed to rule out the presence of an evacuatable mass lesion.

The evaluation of a seizure patient should include blood sugar and serum sodium analyses. Hypoglycemia or hyponatremia (sodium concentration under 120 mEq/L) may cause seizures. The cause of hyponatremia is not always clear but usually includes excessive sodium loss or excessive water intake and may include an excessive, inappropriate antidiuretic hormone secretion. This has been associated with acute and chronic diseases of lung and brain. Young people may develop hyponatremia after vigorous exercise with heavy sweating and repletion of volume with water but not salt. They usually present first with muscle and abdominal cramps but may progress to seizures.

Hypertonic saline treatment is indicated when the serum sodium is below 120 mEq per dl and the patient has shown significant neurologic symptoms. Replacement should be done slowly in order to avoid pulmonary congestion from fluid overload. Other electrolyte abnormalities such as hypocalcemia and hypomagnesemia can cause seizures. Hypomagnesemia is frequently found in alcoholics, and the decision to order serum calcium and magnesium levels is always reasonable in the workup of a new seizure patient.

Needless to say, a blood sugar obtained after giving glucose has little value. A few seconds spent obtaining a sample before therapy would have been worthwhile. Nevertheless, treatment with 50% glucose solution prior to knowing the serum glucose is generally accepted for the acutely obtunded or seizing patient since it virtually never does harm. If the patient has more than a slight probability of being alcoholic, thiamine should be given with or before the first carbohydrate (i.e., glucose) load to prevent Wernicke's encephalopathy.

REFERENCES
Textbook   Rosen. Pp. 1751–1767.

Review Article   Messing, R. O., and Simon, R. P. Seizures as a manifestation of systemic disease. *Neurol. Clin. North Am.* 1986;4:563–584.

Additional   Einser, R. F., et al. Efficacy of a "standard" seizure workup in
References   the emergency department. *Ann. Emerg. Med.* 1986;15:33–
               39.

Joyce, S. M., and Potter, R. Beer potomania: An unusual cause
of symptomatic hyponatremia. *Ann. Emerg. Med.* 1986;15:
745–747.

Case 37 Shaky, Pale, and Drinking

A 35-year-old man had been drinking heavily until two days before he came to the emergency department. When he arrived he complained that he had become shaky and felt sick. He appeared pale, had tremors, and was perspiring but afebrile. The man was alert and gave no evidence of hallucinations. He appeared somewhat dry. He was treated with intravenous fluids and sedation. During the next three hours he began to feel much better and largely lost his tremor. He was discharged, but as he got out of the bed to leave, he collapsed on the floor. He was then found to be hypotensive, and his hematocrit was 13%. Subsequent evaluation showed massive upper gastrointestinal bleeding—probably from a duodenal ulcer or an acute gastritis. The patient was hospitalized for further therapy.

In evaluating a withdrawing alcoholic, what history and physical examination data should be collected to rule out the most common serious associated illnesses?

If you think you are dealing with an upper GI bleeder, what should you do in the ED?

Case 37 was adapted from Platt, F. W., More than DTs. *Emerg. Med.* 1972;4:167.

DISCUSSION   The following workup is very helpful in identifying patients who
are withdrawing from alcohol but are too ill for a simple detoxification (drying-out) facility to handle. The serious diseases
picked up include acute head trauma, acute or chronic subdural
hematomas, epidural hematomas, pneumonia, tuberculosis, GI
bleeding, and severe hypovolemia.

Evaluation of   A. History
Alcohol   1. Chief complaint—main symptom. Duration of symptoms.
Withdrawal   Alleviating and worsening factors. COMMENT: These
Patients   patients often cannot clarify this more than "sick."
                         2. Drinking how much? _____ of what? _____
                            Last drink when? _____ How long this binge? _____
                            When last on detox ward? _____
                         3. Smokes _____ packs/day.
                            Cough _____ oz. _____ (color) sputum/day.
                            Tuberculosis history? _____ Chest pain? _____
                            Short of breath? _____
                         4. Head trauma recently? _____
                            Seizures? _____ Hallucinations? _____
                         5. Vomiting blood? (how much) _____
                            Black, tarry stools? _____
                         6. Taking medications? _____ Allergic to medicines? _____
                            Any other serious illnesses? _____
                         7. Other: _____
                      B. Physical Exam
                         BP _____ P _____ right arm, recumbent
                         BP _____ P _____ right arm, standing or sitting
                                                                (check which)
                         Temp _____ Respiration _____ Weight _____
                         HEENT—(jaundice, evidence of head trauma).
                         Neck, Nodes—
                         Chest—
                         Cardiovascular—(cardiomegaly, edema, gallops, . . .)
                         Abdomen—(tenderness, liver size, . . .)
                         Rectal—Stool to hematest
                         Neurologic—(gait, nystagmus, mental status)
                      C. Lab
                         Chest x-ray _____ CBC _____
                         Urinalysis _____ Blood alcohol _____

Upper GI bleeding is a life-threatening problem. We try to
determine whether the patient is significantly hypovolemic, and
if so expand his blood volume with saline or lactated Ringer's
solution. We pass a nasogastric tube, and if any evidence of
bleeding is obtained, initiate gastric lavage with saline. We ob-

tain blood for typing, crossmatch at least 4 units of whole blood, and do a hematocrit.

Patients with evidence of voluminous blood loss by history or of hypovolemia by examination are admitted, usually to the medical service. Tarry stools or a low hematocrit usually leads to admission. An occasional patient will complain of vomiting blood but will have normal vital signs with no postural change, a normal hematocrit, and negative stool and gastric aspirate. Such a patient may be sent home.

Lower GI bleeding usually presents with red blood passed by rectum. Proctoscopy should be done to locate the bleeding site and evaluate the rectal mucosa. Hemorrhoidal bleeding is, of course, most common and is usually less significant than bleeding from the rectum or higher.

REFERENCES

Textbook

Rosen. Pp. 1423–1430, 2067–2068.

Review Article

Bryson, P. D. *Comprehensive Review in Toxicology.* Rockville, MD, Aspen, 1986. Pp. 141–170.

Additional References

Steer, M. L., and Sile, N. W. Diagnostic procedures in gastrointestinal hemorrhage. *N. Engl. J. Med.* 1983;309:646–650.

Hayashida, M., et al. Comparative effectiveness and cost of inpatient and out-patient detoxification of patients with mild to moderate alcohol withdrawal syndrome. *N. Engl. J. Med.* 1989;320:358–365.

Klerman, G. L. Treatment of alcoholism (editorial). *N. Engl. J. Med.* 1989;320:394–395.

Case 38 Leopard Bite

A 54-year-old zoo keeper was bitten by a leopard. Some sort of illness had killed one leopard in the zoo, and the others were being treated with parenteral tetracycline prophylactically. The zoo keeper was trying to hold the leopard down for its shot when it bit him on the hand. He was seen in the employees' health clinic where he was given a shot of tetanus toxoid. The following day he came to the emergency department complaining of a painful, swollen hand. He was afebrile. There were no red streaks on his arm, and he had only one small, nontender lymph node in the right axilla. Two small, closed puncture wounds were evident. The patient was taken to the operating room where incision and drainage were done under regional anesthesia. Copious pus was drained and cultured.

What organism is most likely to be cultured?

Should the patient be started on rabies vaccine?

Are any other animal bites handled differently?

Is it true that the bite of the leopard is the most dangerous known to humans?

DISCUSSION   Leopards are unusual in having frequent bouts of *Escherichia coli* septicemia. One might thus expect an *E. coli* septic abscess. Nonetheless, the organism cultured was *Pasteurella multocida.* This organism is present in large amounts in the saliva of domestic cats and often in that of dogs. Cat bites are notorious for rapid accumulation of pus and rapid swelling. Fortunately, *P. multocida* is very sensitive to almost any antibiotic and responds well to a ten-day course of penicillin, erythromycin, or tetracycline. With cellulitis one may occasionally do without incision and drainage if the drug is begun before an abscess forms. In this case, initiation of antibiotic therapy one day earlier might have eliminated the need for surgery. It remains controversial whether prophylactic antibiotics given shortly after the time of the bite are effective. Many studies have shown that they are not effective in dog bites, yet prophylactic antibiotics are usually used in both dog and cat bites when the wound is significant. If antibiotics are to be given, then, based on the usual flora, we think reasonable first-line drugs are dicloxacillin in dog bites and penicillin V in cat bites.

Rabies vaccination is not appropriate in this case. The question of rabies prophylaxis usually comes up in connection with a dog bite. Even then, unless there is particular reason for suspicion, no therapy need be done if the animal can be observed. A rabid dog is a sick dog and will either die shortly or be so ill as to warrant sacrificing and autopsy. The city dogcatcher can be notified through the police and will handle the matter. We treat dog bites with copious irrigation, debridement if needed, tetanus toxoid, and antibiotics. We generally suture such wounds, although some do not. When cosmesis is not a consideration, these wounds are probably best left unsutured to freely drain and granulate in. When cosmesis matters, we suggest suturing loosely (to allow for drainage) and giving antibiotics orally. When suturing bites ensure close followup in case an infection develops.

Skunks and bats should be assumed to carry rabies. Other wild mammals may also carry rabies, although for unknown reasons rodents (mice, rats, etc.) almost never do. The local health department is the best resource for determining the potential presence of rabies among the various types of animals in your area. Suspicious bites are treated with rabies immune globulin (half is given into the wound and half intramuscularly) and human diploid cell vaccine (given in five intramuscular injections spread over twenty-eight days). This course of therapy is more effective and less painful than the older, dreaded series of twenty-three injections of duck embryo vaccine into the skin of the abdomen.

Snake bites are benign unless of course the snake is poisonous! Pit vipers (e.g., rattlesnakes) are found throughout most of the United States. These cases will announce themselves by a painful, rapidly developing, local reaction. Treatment is with horse serum antivenin intravenously. Luckily, the only poisonous snake bites in the United States that do not develop such an obvious local reaction are the rarer neurotoxic (elapid) envenomations seen only in zoos (e.g., cobra) or a few isolated parts of the country such as the California desert and the southeast coastal waterways. Serious poisonous arthropod bites are rare in most parts of the country. Black widow spider bites cause painful muscle contractions that can be treated with intravenous calcium. Brown recluse spiders can cause severe local ischemic damage, and their bites are sometimes excised to prevent extensive necrosis. Scorpion stings can cause severe hypertension and anxiety, but most cases are mild except for the stress level of the person bitten.

Human bites are probably the most serious that we see. They should be cleaned, debrided, and copiously irrigated. They must be observed closely and hospitalization urged at any serious sign of infection. Prophylactic antibiotics are appropriate with human bites that "break the skin" (i.e., cause bleeding) and probably should be begun with penicillin.

Hand infections must be aggressively diagnosed and treated to avoid functional disability. Remember that a human "bite" to the metacarpophalangeal joint is often produced by a punch to the mouth. The intra-articular nature of the wound may only be seen if the wound is examined in the fully flexed position, and the patient may not eagerly tell how the metacarpophalangeal joint injury was sustained.

REFERENCES

Textbook   Tintinalli. Pp. 757–765.

Review Article   Callaham, M. Controversies in antibiotic choices for bite wounds. *Ann. Emerg. Med.* 1988;12:1321–1330.

Additional   Galloway, R. E. Mammalian bites. *J. Emerg. Med.* 1988;6:325–
References   331.

                      Kauffman, F. H., and Goldmann, B. J. Rabies. *Am. J. Emerg. Med.* 1986;4:525–531.

Ordog, G. T. The bacteriology of dog bite wounds on initial presentation. *Ann. Emerg. Med.* 1986;15:1324–1329.

Curry, S. C., et al. The legitimacy of rattlesnake bites in Central Arizona. *Ann. Emerg. Med.* 1989;18:658–663.

Case 39 Coma

A 50-year-old man was brought to the emergency department by ambulance. He had been found lying in the street unconscious. There was no obvious evidence of trauma.

On arrival the man was comatose. He appeared unkempt, unshaven, and dirty. There was a distinct alcohol odor mingled with several less well-defined odors. He moved away from painful stimuli but would not respond to verbal communications. Vital signs included a pulse rate of 100, respiratory rate of 15, blood pressure of 160/90, and temperature of 37.5°C rectally. He had positive oculocephalic reflexes, commonly termed "doll's eyes" (on tilting his head to the right, his eyes briefly moved to the left, and vice versa). His muscle tone was normal throughout. Deep tendon reflexes were symmetric, although ankle jerks could not be elicited. The plantar responses were flexor. Respiration was regular. There was no evidence of head trauma, and pupils were equal. An intravenous route was established, and 50 ml of 50% glucose solution was given. No response was noted. The patient was thought to be in alcoholic stupor. Blood sugar, electrolyte, and blood alcohol analyses were ordered. The patient was laid flat on his back, tied with gauze restraints, and left to sober up. Two hours later he vomited and aspirated some of the vomitus. He did not suffer a respiratory arrest but was thought to have an aspiration pneumonitis and was admitted to the medical ward.

What is the preferred position in which to place comatose patients?

How do you treat aspiration?

DISCUSSION   Coma position should ensure patency of the airway. If the patient vomits (not uncommon in an unconscious patient), the emesis should be able to pour out by gravity and not remain in the pharynx to cause obstruction or be aspirated into the lungs. The standard position is semiprone, semilateral decubitus with the mouth pointed down near the edge of the bed. Vomitus will then tend to pour off the bed. The patient can be tied in such a position and be relatively safe.

Of course, nothing is better than close observation, but all too often a patient is well observed in an ED until a patient in worse shape arrives, and then attention is diverted from the first patient. Some emergency units have attached observation wards with monitoring facilities and a separate nursing staff. Even when such an intensive care observation unit is maintained, observation may be inadequate when the system becomes overloaded.

Observation should include looking for signs of increasing intracranial pressure (checking for arousability, pulse, blood pressure, and pupillary size and reactivity). A comatose patient who is not clearly more alert in four hours should be admitted to the hospital.

Coma is an emergency with metabolic, toxicologic, and neurologic causes. A history of trauma or the presence of an asymmetric neurologic deficit suggests a mass lesion such as a subdural or epidural hematoma. Venous blood sampling may reveal hypoglycemia, hyperglycemia, hepatic or renal failure, or ethanol or other toxic ingestion. Arterial blood sampling may reveal an unsuspected metabolic acidoses (from shock or poison) or hypoxia.

When presented with a comatose patient, it is necessary to act before all the data (e.g., blood tests) are back. All coma patients should promptly be given oxygen, 25 gm of glucose, 0.8 mg or more of Narcan, and 50 to 100 mg of thiamine. This empiric therapy should be given unless the cause of unconsciousness is clear. A complete neurologic examination must be performed on all comatose patients. This includes pupillary size and reactivity, best motor response, deep tendon reflexes, and checking for the presence of an abnormal Babinski response. Any lateralizing neurologic signs mandate an emergency head computed tomogram, as does an unexpectedly prolonged unconscious state (e.g., a seizure patient who does not wake up).

Once a patient has aspirated, severe chemical pneumonitis may develop. Steroids are no longer used for treatment of aspiration pneumonitis. Antibiotics should be used if signs of infection, such as fever and purulent sputum, develop.

REFERENCES
Textbook   Rosen. Pp. 249–267.

Review Article   Ropper, A. H., and Martin, J. B. Coma and Other Disorders of
                        Consciousness. In E. Braunwald et al. (eds.), *Harrison's Prin-
                        ciples of Internal Medicine* (11th edition). New York, McGraw-
                        Hill, 1987. Pp. 114–120.

Additional   Pennza, T. T. Aspiration pneumonia, necrotizing pneumonia,
Reference   and lung abscess. *Emerg. Med. Clin. North Am.* 1989;7:279–
                        307.

Case 40 Coughing Up Blood

A 23-year-old man came to the emergency department complaining of shortness of breath, fatigue, and coughing up blood. He claimed he had had these symptoms for about ten months and denied any remarkable recent worsening. He admitted smoking one pack of cigarettes daily. His cough produced about 1 ounce of almost pure blood daily. He could do very little without dyspnea and had quit his job about one year earlier because of fatigue and dyspnea. He slept flat but several times a week awoke with choking and walked about the house, drank water, even went outdoors before settling back in bed. He denied any chest pain and had no history of rheumatic fever or heart murmur.

This night he called for help when he awoke from an afternoon nap in a state of panic. He was confused and terrified. The confusion quickly disappeared, but the panic remained. He had recently been having marital difficulties and was separated from his wife. In the past there had been several episodes of panic but none as severe as this day's.

On physical examination, the patient appeared anxious and tremulous. His pulse was 100, respiration 24, blood pressure 150/80, and temperature 37.5° C. His chest was clear, jugular venous pressure was normal, and he had no edema. Pulses were normal. His cardiac impulse was forceful but not sustained and was localized at the fourth intercostal space in the midclavicular line. He had no abnormal gallops, a loud S_1 and S_2, and a faint short systolic murmur at the aortic area. On being asked to cough, he produced bloody saliva by sucking at a bleeding gum about a carious tooth. He had no adenopathy and no thyromegaly. The patient appeared otherwise normal. A chest x-ray was normal.

What should next be done for this patient?

In what order should organic and psychiatric symptoms be pursued in the ED?

DISCUSSION   This young man presented clear organic-sounding symptoms and clear emotional symptoms. Of the two, the reason for this arrival at the ED was acute panic, and this should be addressed. Physicians are often loath to approach psychiatric problems due to their own insecurities. Nonetheless, the ED must attend primarily to the problems bringing the patient to the hospital. Often, as in this case, a combined approach works best.

This man was assured that he had several problems, that his lungs and heart seemed to have nothing seriously wrong with them but that he should be seen in the medical clinic. He was told that an interview with one of the psychiatric staff was essential, after which he was given some mild sedation (Valium, 5 mg, two to four times a day). After the initial psychiatric interview, the patient was calmer and returned home.

This case was grossly unfinished as the patient left the ED; however, several things were begun. An appraisal had been made of possible life-threatening cardiac or pulmonary disease and none found. The importance of the emotional features of the illness had been stressed to the patient and arrangements made for followup. The obvious features of malingering (sucking on a bleeding mouth lesion and claiming the bloody saliva as hemoptysis) did not go unnoticed, but the patient properly was not punished for this. In fact, this unusual behavior should be viewed as a cry for help—producing more symptoms in order to be heard.

In general, one should work up what appears to be most prominent. A barber once told me that his technique was "to cut off whatever sticks out." This is the most fruitful ED approach—that is, examine whatever sticks out. If psychopathology stares you in the face, evaluate it first, not after a major organic workup proves negative. Fear of labeling the patient a neurotic should not lead the doctor to avoid dealing with emotional symptoms that the patient desperately wants to discuss.

Hemoptysis can be an acute medical emergency when massive, but more frequently presents as small amounts of blood-tinged sputum such as with tracheobronchitis. A complete examination should rule out malignancy, pneumonia, hypertension, and mitral stenosis as the cause.

Benzodiazepines are useful agents for the treatment of acute anxiety, but must only be used for short periods until proper medical and psychiatric followup can be arranged. The importance of psychiatric evaluation must be stressed to the patient before the underlying emotional problems can be addressed and corrected. The evaluation in the ED must include an assessment of suicide potential.

REFERENCES

Textbook   Schwartz. Pp. 740–745.

Review Article   Goldmann, J. M. Hemoptysis: Emergency assessment and management. *Emerg. Med. Clin. North Am.* 1989;7:325–337.

Additional   O'Shea, B., et al. Factitious hemoptysis. *Arch. Intern. Med.*
References   1984;144(2) 415–419.

                        Rudzinski, J. P., and delCasciall, J. Massive hemoptysis. *Ann. Emerg. Med.* 1987;16:1561–1564.

Case 41 Repeat Visits

A 20-year-old woman was brought to the emergency department on a Saturday night with a laceration. She had cut herself with a razor blade and was brought in by ambulance. The EMT had placed a pressure dressing on her superficial wrist laceration, which was bleeding slowly. The patient was relatively uncommunicative but admitted she felt depressed.

During the preceding eighteen months the woman had spent over thirteen months hospitalized on several psychiatric wards with the diagnosis of depression. During the preceding week she had appeared at the ED five times. She had been discharged from the psychiatry inpatient unit on Tuesday and that same evening returned to the ED with slashed wrists. The wounds were irrigated and sutured, and she was referred to the psychiatry team, who interviewed her and judged her to be not suicidal. Two days later, on Thursday, she arrived at the ED to discuss her worsening depression with the psychiatry team. After her interview she went out, only to return four hours later with a new laceration of the left wrist. On Friday she was brought in with a presumed overdose of aspirin, Librium, and Thorazine. She refused to wait for a physician to see her and left within an hour of her arrival. The ED had been very busy with major trauma cases, and both nurses and physicians viewed her as a nuisance rather than as a challenging new problem. On Saturday night she returned with her latest laceration. She was again sutured and referred to the psychiatry team. She announced that she was now under the care of an outside private psychiatrist. When he was called, he responded by stating that she was no suicide risk and that he was getting disgusted with her. Her parents had both killed themselves when she was 3 years old.

Is this patient suicidal?

One of the physicians claims that the patient is in the running for the "Turkey of the Year Award." How do you believe she should be handled?

DISCUSSION   All patients who have taken an overdose, made a suicidal gesture, made threats against themselves or others, are intoxicated,
or wish to sign out of the ED against medical advice must have
a careful mental status examination performed. This should include orientation to person, place, time, content of thought, and
the presence of hallucinations or suicidal or homicidal ideations.
(Patients who have hallucinations that consist of commands of
any sort are at the highest risk for suicidal or homicidal actions
and usually should be hospitalized in a psychiatric facility.) Abnormalities should be carefully documented on the medical record for serial examinations. Any potentially suicidal patients
and acutely psychotic patients should be seen by a psychiatrist
prior to leaving the ED. Intoxicated patients should be held in
the department until they have "sobered up" unless they are
taken home by another responsible person. Patients in these
categories who are allowed to leave without proper supervision
represent a threat to themselves and a risk of malpractice suit
against the ED staff for negligence in allowing them to leave.

A successful suicide is by definition a disastrous event. In
general, when a patient admits to depression, she should be
queried about suicidal thoughts or plans. These should be taken
seriously. Viewing the gamut of patients who have made a suicide attempt and failed, one finds some with serious depression
and desire to kill themselves and others with far less emotional
distress who intended a mere gesture or an appeal for help,
love, attention, or even punishment. Unfortunately serious in-
tent does not always ensure success, and a mere gesture may
accidentally be fatal. In general, psychiatrists tend to put the
most effort into aiding suicidally depressed patients and not into
working with persons they judge to be immature gesturers. This
patient may die by her own hand eventually, but any one attempt is not likely to be a serious one.

This patient exemplifies an extremely difficult ED problem. It
is not clear what she is getting from the ED, but it is hard to
believe that she is in any way getting assistance. She has been
labeled a "chronic underdoser." Her diagnosis is probably "borderline personality disorder," and she will continue to be very
difficult for therapists of any sort. Harassing the staff seems to
be part of a destructive game she plays, destructive to her and
to those superficially appearing to help her. At the very least,
she is crying wolf too often and probably will not be heard
when she cries the last time. She is becoming the victim of
considerable ED staff hostility—perhaps indeed what she is trying to provoke. She interrupts and dilutes the care of other

patients and makes the staff aware of its abject failure in dealing with her.

No one has been able to find a satisfactory approach to this sort of patient. She is a depressed lost soul with no hope, and few successes. She does almost nothing well, not even suicide attempts, and her more or less pathologic involvement with the ED may be all the human contact she can tolerate or obtain. An apocryphal tale says that for a similar patient a collection was taken up one night by the ED staff. The collection bought a one-way bus ticket to a city 600 miles away and temporarily stopped the patient's visits. A more constructive approach for these patients is to involve staff from the ED, psychiatry, and social services in a meeting to work out an individualized patient treatment plan. In selected cases, we have had some success with this type of interagency team approach, at least in the short term.

REFERENCES
Textbook   Rosen. Pp. 1835–1844.

Review Article   Clayton, P. J. Suicide. *Psychiatr. Clin. North Am.* 1985;8:203–214.

Additional   Ruben, H. L. Managing suicidal behavior. *J.A.M.A.* 1979;241:
References   282–284.

Bhatia, S. C., et al. Suicide risk: Evaluation and management. *Am. Fam. Physician* 1986;34:167–174.

Case 42 Seventy-Two Years Old, Feeling Faint

A 72-year-old man was brought to the emergency department because he had become faint at a bowling alley. On arrival at the ED he felt well. He was placed in the cardiac resuscitation room because that night it possessed the only working ECG. On examination he denied faintness, shortness of breath, or chest pain. He was being cared for by an outside physician and was on no medications. He believed that he had had a "heart attack" five years earlier that consisted of "auricular fibrillation."

His blood pressure was 110/70. His pulse was counted at 104 and was noted to be irregular; an apical pulse of 120 was noted. He had no edema, rales, or elevation of jugular venous pressure. He had carotid bruits but no heart murmurs. The diagnostic ECG was normal except for the presence of atrial fibrillation.

While the patient was resting, still attached to the ECG monitor, he noted an unusual formation on the monitor oscilloscope and called it to the attention of the physician and nurse in the room. The formation appeared to be five ventricular beats in a row. These ended spontaneously and did not reappear. A defibrillator paddle was coated with electrode paste and placed under the patient's upper back. The other paddle was coated, and the capacitor charged with 200 watt seconds. An intravenous injection of lidocaine, 100 mg, was given. The patient's physician was contacted. He agreed to take over the patient's care if he could be transferred to a nearby private hospital but questioned the wisdom of moving him at that time.

Did this patient have a run of ventricular tachycardia?

How do you treat ventricular tachycardia?

What might have led to this patient's arrhythmias?

DISCUSSION   Ventricular tachycardia (VT) is usually a life-threatening arrhythmia because of the likelihood of its proceeding to ventricu-
lar fibrillation. In the ED it should always be assumed to be a
disastrous arrhythmia and not the "benign ventricular tachycardia" that is often noted in coronary care units. Treatment
should be rapid.

If the blood pressure seems adequate, testifying to a reasonable cardiac output, a bolus of lidocaine 1 mg per kg should be
given. Additional lidocaine may be given, up to a total of 3 mg
per kg or until the arrhythmia subsides. If the maximum permis-
sible dose has been given and the VT persists, procainamide
(Pronestyl) can be tried next. If the arrhythmia persists, cardioversion should be employed. In the unstable patient with chest
pain, dyspnea, or hypotension, synchronized cardioversion starting at 50 joules is the first treatment of choice. If time permits,
some form of analgesia/sedation should be employed prior to
the cardioversion. In the patient with pulseless VT and wit-
nessed arrest, a precardial thump is delivered, and if unsuccessful, defibrillation is started at 200 joules. More energy is given if
needed; up to 360 joules if the initial shock is not successful. If
the arrhythmia persists, cardiopulmonary resuscitation is begun, followed by intravenous epinephrine (0.5 to 1.0 mg), intubation, and repeated attempts at defibrillation at 360 joules. If
unsuccessful, lidocaine is given followed by defibrillation. If this
is unsuccessful, bretylium may be used.

In this case the patient converted spontaneously after a brief
run of five ventricular beats. One could question whether five
beats make a ventricular tachycardia, but a more important
question is whether this was indeed VT or just aberration of
conduction through the ventricles from a supraventricular tachycardia. Normally one can tell a supraventricular tachycardia
from VT simply by the width of the QRS. In some cases when
there is aberrant conduction through the ventricle of the supraventricular beat, the QRS is widened. Even a cardiologist with
plenty of time to study the tracing may have trouble differentiating a VT from a supraventricular tachycardia with aberrancy.
In this case the absence of a written record to study makes
things even more difficult, and it is not wise to observe a patient
too long to secure evidence that may be diagnostic for the
physician but lethal for the patient. Lidocaine should be given
here intravenously in a 100-mg bolus and followed by a lidocaine drip at 2 to 4 mg per minute.

Patients with myocardial infarctions may or may not have
serious arrhythmias. On the other hand, a patient with life-

threatening arrhythmias may not have had an infarction even though he has atherosclerotic coronary artery disease. Coronary artery disease may present with sudden death, myocardial infarction, self-limiting or benign arrhythmias, congestive heart failure, or angina pectoris. These may occur in combination or singly. With no clear history of pain or an ECG diagnostic of infarction, we cannot yet say whether this patient had a myocardial infarction; however, he surely should be hospitalized. His atrial fibrillation may be a recent change and may be responsible for his faintness. He may have had a brief but more serious arrhythmia at the bowling alley. His blood pressure is probably low and may be related to the arrhythmia or to the cause of the arrhythmia. Pulmonary embolism should be searched for as a cause of the atrial fibrillation. If this patient has been on digitalis, digitoxicity should be considered as another possible cause of his various arrhythmias.

Transportation to another hospital should not be done at this time due to the inherent instability of the patient's situation. The emergency physician caring for the patient is responsible for making sure the patient is stable for transport. In fact, the emergency physician is responsible for care delivered (or not delivered) en route and until the patient is seen by the physician at the receiving facility.

The fact that this patient diagnosed his own ventricular tachycardia should not lessen its serious import for us. We should be doing the monitoring and should not have to rely on the patient to do this. At no time should his monitoring be unattended, from arrival in the ED to the coronary care unit.

REFERENCES

Textbook   Rosen. Pp. 104–105, 1259–1278.

Review Article Stapczynski, J. S., and Podrid, P. J. Coping with the vagaries of ventricular ectopy. *Emerg. Med. Rep.* 1989;10:(3)17–24.

Additional References Baerman, J. M., et al. Differentiation of ventricular tachycardia from supraventricular tachycardia with aberration: Value of the clinical history. *Ann. Emerg. Med.* 1987;16:40–43.

Levitt, M. A. Supraventricular tachycardia with aberrant conduction vs. ventricular tachycardia: Differentiation and diagnosis. *Am. J. Emerg. Med.* 1988;6:273–277.

Case **43** Falling Down Stairs

A 44-year-old man came to the emergency department complaining of chest pain after a fall down stairs four hours earlier while going to work. He had begun to hurt then, and the pain was worst at the right lower rib cage. He also hurt over the right buttock, where he had bounced down several steps. He noted pain in his chest on breathing deeply. He had smoked about one pack of cigarettes daily for about thirty years and always had a morning cough. Alcohol intake was not commented on.

On physical examination, the patient had marked tenderness over the right fifth through tenth ribs, maximal in the midaxillary line. His chest was clear to auscultation. He was afebrile, and otherwise normal.

X-ray pictures were taken, and no hip fracture or pulmonary infiltrates were seen. The patient had several lateral rib fractures. After his chest was painted with benzoin, 3-inch adhesive tape was applied from past the anterior midline around the painful hemithorax to a point past the vertebrae posteriorly. The tape was applied in overlapping strips to cover the hemithorax from the fourth to the eleventh ribs. The patient was given twenty tablets of acetaminophen with ½ grain of codeine and told to take one every four hours as needed for pain. He felt much better after the taping and thanked the physician.

Two days later the patient returned with more pain and a fever. Examination showed decreased breath sounds, rales, and wheezes at the right lung base. His temperature was 38.0° orally. A chest x-ray showed an extensive right lower lobe pneumonia. He was admitted to the hospital for therapy.

Was the pneumonia an obligatory complication of the rib fractures?

What should have been done differently?

DISCUSSION   Rib fracture should be suspected if sharp pain that increases with cough or deep breathing develops after trauma or a heavy cough. The diagnosis can be made clinically, and in simple cases confirmation by rib x-rays is unnecessary since rib bruises and rib fractures are treated similarly. We do recommend taking a standard PA and lateral chest x-ray to rule out hemothorax, pneumothorax, pulmonary contusion, or pathologic fracture from metastatic disease. Most rib fractures will be seen on these films. If no fracture is seen, we tell patients that we believe they may have a fractured rib and treat them for it. We explain that if the injury is only a contusion, they will be better sooner.

An effective cough, an effective mucociliary apparatus, and adequate local ventilation are all parts of maintaining the health of the lung. When these three mechanisms or other resistance phenomena are subverted, pneumonia is more likely. Smokers have considerable suppression of the ciliary activity in their bronchi and may not clear bacteria and debris from the lungs in the usual fashion. A cough may be essential. Codeine suppresses cough easily and may have been instrumental in the pneumonia development. The splinting induced by pain may be considerable, but taping adds to this and decreases local ventilation. This patient should have been urged to stop smoking and instructed in deep-breathing exercises. Patient compliance will not be good unless adequate analgesia is prescribed.

The pneumonia rate is high in smokers who have fractured ribs, and the pain problem is difficult to deal with. This patient's alcohol intake was not discussed with him. Alcohol suppresses host defenses in several ways, including suppression of the bone marrow resulting in leukopenia and suppression of the pulmonary mucociliary apparatus. If he was indeed a drinker, he should have been urged to abstain after his rib fractures. Finally, the actual fall down stairs was not defined clearly enough. Why and how did he fall down stairs? Had he been faint? Dizzy? Drunk? The event before the event bringing him to the ED (the fall) may be the most important part of his illness, and patients like this should be questioned about syncope, vertigo, dizziness, or light-headedness. This may prompt further workup.

"Prophylactic" antibiotic therapy might be used in this sort of case to treat the bronchitis and avoid the development of pneumonia.

REFERENCES
Textbook   Rosen. Pp. 473–478.

Review Article   Atkins, P. C., Corso, P. J., and Laurance Hill J. Chest Wall
                        Trauma. In C. Dewitt and M. D. Daughtry (eds.), *Thoracic
                        Trauma*. Boston, Little Brown, 1980. Pp. 39–51.

Additional   Thompson, B. N., et al. Rib radiographs for trauma: Useful or
Reference   wasteful? *Ann. Emerg. Med.* 1986;15:261–265.

Case 44 Probably Drunk

A 30-year-old man was brought to the emergency department by ambulance. He was described by the EMT as confused and probably drunk. He was noted to be absent without leave from a local private psychiatric hospital where he had been treated for alcoholism and had been on disulfiram (Antabuse) for one week. Today he had left the hospital and had drunk 1 quart of wine. Feeling ill, he went to a nearby police car and asked for assistance.

On arrival at the ED, the patient was observed to be uncooperative and lobster red in color, and he had a tachycardia of 140 beats per minute with a systolic blood pressure of 70 mm Hg. His chest was clear; his heart seemed normal except for the tachycardia; and he seemed otherwise normal. Rectal exam revealed brown stool that was negative when tested for occult blood. There was no obvious evidence of trauma. His jugular venous pressure seemed normal or low. His skin was warm and dry.

He was given 2000 ml of normal saline solution intravenously over sixty minutes. A chest x-ray and an ECG were done; they were normal. One gram of ascorbic acid (vitamin C) was given intravenously, and the patient lost his flush. The blood pressure moved up to 110 systolic by the end of his first liter of intravenous fluids. He left the ED four hours later feeling much better.

What causes hypotension in the alcohol-Antabuse reaction?

How should it be treated?

What does the vitamin C do?

DISCUSSION   Hypotension is a cardinal sign of a serious disease state and
should be attacked vigorously. To do so one needs certain parameters and some of these were not obtained in this case.
Most important are blood pressure, temperature, pulse, an estimate of the central venous pressure, weight, hematocrit, BUN,
urine output, and serum sodium levels. With these one can
attempt to distinguish among the three main mechanisms of
hypotension and monitor treatment. Cardiogenic shock usually
is accompanied by an elevation of the venous pressure. Of
course hypotension from any cause may lead to insufficient
coronary artery perfusion and secondary pump failure. Hypovolemia due to bleeding (into fracture sites, the gastrointestinal
tract, the peritoneum, retroperitoneum, chest cavity, or externally) will lead to hypotension when about 30% of the blood
volume is lost. Water and salt may be lost externally or simply
moved out of the vascular compartment, as is thought to be the
case in alcohol-Antabuse reactions. Finally, vascular collapse
due to adrenal insufficiency, sepsis, hypoxia, or drugs can lead
to hypotension. Treatment of vascular collapse or hypovolemia
is similar—rapid infusions of large amounts of crystalloids, colloid, or blood. A solution of 5% dextrose in water is a poor fluid
for this purpose, and we usually start with normal saline solution or lactated Ringer's solution.

Antabuse interferes with the metabolism of alcohol in the
same way that metronidazole (Flagyl) can. They cause a pile-up
of acetaldehyde, presumably by blocking the enzyme acetaldehyde dehydrogenase. Acetaldehyde can mimic some of the features of the alcohol-Antabuse reaction but *not* the hypotension,
so it is not in itself enough to explain the reaction. The additional effect may be caused by a breakdown product of Antabuse
that interferes with catecholamine metabolism. The profound
shock that results from these combined effects may be resistant
to all catechols except intravenous norepinephrine. As little as 7
ml of alcohol can produce the syndrome.

The reasons for use of vitamin C are obscure, but it seems to
lessen the symptoms of the alcohol-Antabuse reaction. Some
alcoholics even take oral vitamin C to "counteract the Antabuse" before drinking.

Drug reactions should always be considered in the differential
diagnosis of patients who are on any medications. Many mild
reactions result from common medications (such as aspirin
leading to asymptomatic gastrointestinal bleeding or diuretics
leading to generalized mild weakness). There are also a number
of rarer or obscure but potentially lethal reactions, such as mix-

ing Demerol (meperidine) and a MAO inhibitor, or Antabuse and ethanol.

REFERENCES

Textbook   Rosen. Pp. 2079–2080.

Review Article   Motte, S., et al. Refractory hyperdynamic shock associated with alcohol and disulfiram. *Am. J. Emerg. Med.* 1986;4:323–325.

Additional   Saxe, T. G. Drug-alcohol interactions. *Am. Fam. Phys.* 1986;
Reference   33:159–162.

Case 45 Pain on Urination

A 54-year-old woman came to the emergency department complaining of pain on urination over a period of several hours. She was urinating almost every thirty minutes and noted that her urine had become red. She had had many past episodes of similar suprapubic and low back pain with passage of urine. A total abdominal hysterectomy had been done ten years earlier for "pelvic relaxation." Cystoscopy had been done five years earlier with a diagnosis of trigonitis but no evidence of obstruction. Several intravenous pyelograms (IVPs) had been done in the past and were normal.

On physical examination the patient was observed to be obese; she had a blood pressure of 174/110 and a temperature of 37.5°C orally. There was no costovertebral angle tenderness, and her abdomen was normal. No rectal or pelvic examination was done.

A urinalysis showed 2+ protein, over 50 red blood cells (RBCs) and over 50 white blood cells (WBCs) per high-power field of spun sediment. A urine culture was done and later showed over 100,000 colonies of *Escherichia coli* per milliliter. All antibiotics tested were effective against the organism in vitro. The diagnosis then considered was hemorrhagic cystitis. She was placed on ampicillin, 500 mg orally qid for ten days, and pyridium, 100 mg tid for three days. Another IVP was scheduled and done the next day. It was normal. The patient was referred to the urology clinic. Despite her referral, she returned to the ED ten days after her first visit, now complaining of back pain and chills. She admitted to not taking her ampicillin regularly. She was afebrile but now had left flank tenderness. Her repeat urinalysis showed about 4 RBCs and WBCs per high-power field; there was no more proteinuria. She was given more ampicillin and urged to take it as directed.

What is the most common reason for failure of drug therapy?

How should followup care be arranged for patients with urinary tract infections?

152

When should an IVP be done in patients with urinary tract symptoms?

What is a significant white blood cell count in a urinalysis?

DISCUSSION   It should not be surprising that the primary reason drug therapy fails is the patient's failure to take the drug. Many patients will do poorly at following directions when given only one drug, and the failure rate goes up as the number of prescriptions given increases. In general, one should try to limit therapy to a single drug. If several drugs or procedures are being advised, one should clearly define expectations and plans for the patient. The patient should understand why the drug was prescribed, how it is to be taken, its significant side effects, and when to expect resolution of symptoms. It must be clear that she understands the plan, and that is best achieved by providing the patient with a legible discharge instruction sheet written in plain English in addition to a verbal communication. You know that your message has been communicated if the patient can recite it back to you.

Most patients who present with urinary tract symptoms at the ED have disease limited to the urethra or bladder. The question of which urinary tract infection (UTI) patients need a urine culture remains controversial. Some think that cultures need not be done in a woman with an apparently benign case of cystitis, but others believe that all patients with suspected UTI deserve a urine culture since it is so confusing when a patient's symptoms fail to resolve on therapy and she had no culture initially. Symptomatic UTIs often fail to produce more than 100,000 organisms per ml on culture, and if a woman is symptomatic with pyuria, we consider a clean-catch culture to be positive if there are more than 10,000 per ml, especially if there is only one organism. The standard treatment for cystitis used to be a ten-day course of sulfa, tetracycline, or ampicillin. Clinical research over the past several years has demonstrated that seven-, five-, or three-day courses or even a single dose with any of a variety of antibiotics may be effective. The most effective of the single-dose regimens is trimethoprim/sulfamethoxazole (two double-strength tablets).

If the antibiotic is appropriate, the pyuria or hematuria should be nearly cleared in two days, and the dysuria should be gone in twenty-four hours. Repeat urinalysis should be done two to three days after conclusion of antibiotic therapy.

A surprising number (perhaps 20%) have some pyuria but no bacilluria and recover with or without antibiotics in the same three to seven days.

Any evidence of renal involvement in a UTI (such as flank pain, high fever, or costovertebral angle tenderness) suggests acute pyelonephritis, a form of acute interstitial nephritis due to infection that produces a septic picture with fever, chills, flank pain, nausea, tachycardia, and malaise. Signs of cystitis, leukocyte casts, and bacteria in unspun clean-catch urine samples may also be seen. As with most clinical syndromes, not all these signs and symptoms need be present in any one patient. Patients who are toxic should be placed on parenteral antibiotics and admitted. Any patient who is less sick, is able to keep down fluids, and has no underlying disease such as diabetes may be treated as an outpatient if close followup and home support are available. Any evidence of obstruction warrants an emergency IVP.

An IVP with postvoiding films should also be done as part of a urologic workup in cases of repeated UTI. We usually work up a male with his second infection and a female with her third. Cystoscopy is appropriate at this stage, and so a referral to a urologist is needed. If gross hematuria is present, referral is best even with a "first infection."

It is not clear how much leukocytosis in the urine constitutes pyuria. Women may have several WBCs per high-power field with no infection, but in men even a few WBCs may be significant.

Recurrent urethritis or cystitis in postmenopausal women may be associated with atrophic vaginal mucosa due to estrogen lack. Treatment with estrogens improves the status of vaginal and urethral mucosa and decreases the incidence of infections. The full effects of this treatment in terms of possibly inducing some types of cancer and protecting against others are still being looked into.

REFERENCES

Textbook   Tintinalli. Pp. 361–365.

Review Article   Shea, D. G. Pyelonephritis and female urinary tract infection. *Emerg. Med. Clin. North Am.* 1988;6:403–417.

Additional   Werman, H. A., and Brown, C. G. Utility of the urine cultures
References   in the emergency department. *Ann. Emerg. Med.* 1986;15:302–307.

               Block, B. Urinary tract infections. *Am. Fam. Physician* 1986;6: 172–185.

Case 46 Mental Status: Confused

A 50-year-old woman was brought to the emergency department by paramedics. On arrival, they stated that she had been found by her landlady lethargic and confused. The landlady had been concerned about the patient because she had not seen her in the previous two days—an unusual occurrence.

The EMTs said that at the scene they found one hypertensive medication, although they "did not have time to look real well" for other pill bottles.

Her initial blood pressure at the scene was 230/140. The patient was described at that time as incoherent and generally lethargic with periods of combativeness.

On preliminary exam the ED physician found a mildly obese female making "nonsense statements" but moving all extremities. She had periods of thrashing about on the stretcher. She was breathing at a rate of 20 without apparent difficulty. Her pulse was 70, her temperature 96.5 rectally, and her blood pressure in the ED was 250/140.

The heart/lung exam revealed fine rales at the bases and an S3 gallop. She had blurred optic disc margins with anteriolar narrowing and bilateral hemorrhages and exudate.

The neurologic exam revealed bilateral extensor response of the great toes. No other focal abnormality was noted.

When dealing with hypertensive disease syndromes, how does one gauge the relative severity of the initial presentation?

What initial treatment regimens would have been appropriate in this case?

DISCUSSION   Much confusion exists concerning the treatment of patients with acute elevation of blood pressure. When treating such patients, it is crucial to be neither overly cautious nor overly aggressive. Too little therapy can result in life-threatening end-organ dysfunction of the central nervous system, heart, or kidneys; too much therapy can also threaten those same organs by diminishing their blood flow.

One useful method of categorizing acute hypertensive syndromes is to define them as being either a hypertensive emergency or a hypertensive urgency.

In cases of *hypertensive emergencies,* the diastolic blood pressure is usually 135 or greater, and evidence exists of significant dysfunction of the central nervous system, heart, or kidneys. Obviously, the physical exam, a mental status exam, a serum BUN level, and a routine urine analysis are critically important in making this categorization. Funduscopic and neurologic exams may reveal papilledema or focal deficits, or the heart and lung exams may show signs of congestive heart failure. The patient's mental status exam is always abnormal in cases of hypertensive emergency. To quickly assess the patient's mental status, one should determine if she is alert and oriented to person, place, and time. If not, does she respond appropriately to verbal or painful stimuli, or is she unresponsive?

Patients may present with less severe manifestations of hypertensive disease, often termed *hypertensive urgency,* in which the diastolic blood pressure is generally less than 130, and end-organ dysfunction, particularly of the central nervous system, is absent or very mild. In these cases, emergency therapy, i.e., therapy within the first hour, is generally not critical.

Clearly this patient's clinical presentation is that of an hypertensive emergency given her alteration in mental status, retinopathy, and evidence of congestive heart failure. In addition, her diastolic blood pressure is 140; therefore, it is very important in this particular patient to initiate therapy quickly but cautiously to limit morbidity and mortality. Current standards suggest that the diastolic blood pressure should not be lowered below 105 in the initial treatment phase. The fear of lowering the blood pressure too much with subsequent underperfusion of vital organs is a real one, and careful monitoring of blood pressure at all times is mandatory.

Many pharmacologic agents are available to treat patients with hypertensive emergencies. Sodium nitroprusside is presently the single best agent, but it must be used with great caution and with careful monitoring. Labetalol (an alpha- and beta-blocking agent), nifedipine (a calcium channel blocker), and loop diuretics are second-line agents that may also be useful in treating these emergencies. A useful method of gently lowering an elevated pressure in a patient without altered mental status or congestive heart failure is with a single sublingual dose of nifedipine. This is a common, although not currently an FDA approved, use of this drug.

REFERENCES
Textbook   Tintinalli. Pp. 222–231.

Review Article   Reuler, J. B., and Magarian, G. J. Hypertensive emergency and urgency. *J. Gen. Intern. Med.* 1988;3:64–74.

Additional   Catapno, M. S., and Marx, J. A. Management of urgent hyper-
References   tension: A comparison of oral treatment regimens in the emergency department. *J. Emerg. Med.* 1986;4:361–368.

                     Ellrodt, A. G., and Ault, M. J. Calcium channel blockers in acute hypertension. *Am. J. Emerg. Med.* 1985;3(6 Suppl.):16–24.

Case 47 Seeing Zebras

A 38-year-old woman was taken to another hospital's emergency department by concerned relatives. She stated that she awoke in the morning and saw two strange men in her house. She called the police, but the men mysteriously disappeared. Later there were "several zebras walking across the wall." Her son stated that she was a heavy drinker and that she drank to keep from being nervous.

On physical examination the patient was noted to have a tachycardia (120) but to be afebrile. Her blood pressure was 114/90. She was anxious and tachypneic but well oriented. Reflexes were brisk and pupils dilated but reactive. She complained of thirst and a dry mouth. The ED doctor at the time, a retired surgeon, gave her 100 mg of Librium intramuscularly and then called a medical resident to see her. The second doctor noted that she had a peripheral neuropathy. His diagnoses were (1) delirium tremens (DTs), (2) alcoholic myopathy and neuropathy, and (3) depression. She was referred to our ED for admission to the alcohol detoxification unit.

On arrival at our ED the woman denied much recent drinking. Her blood pressure was 100/70 supine and 80/65 sitting, and her pulse was 120 sitting. A hematocrit was 42% and stool hematest negative. She said she really did not want to go to the detoxification ward—she did not consider herself to be an alcoholic. The staff physician seeing her pointed out that not everyone in the ED that day was hallucinating, and the sooner she realized she was an alcoholic the sooner she might be able to do something about it.

Samples were drawn for complete blood count, electrolytes, BUN, sugar, biochemical survey, VDRL, and blood alcohol analyses; and urinalysis and chest x-rays were done. The patient was admitted to the alcohol detoxification unit, and ten minutes later the electrolytes were reported to be Na 118, Cl 83, HCO$_3$ 9, and K 2.8 mEq/L. Alcohol level was only 27 mg per 100 milliliters. A phone call to the woman's relatives uncovered the fact that she had indeed been depressed and probably had taken an overdose of aspirin and an over-the-counter sedative containing scopolamine. Serum salicylate level was 47 mg per 100 milliliters, several times the normal therapeutic level.

Did the patient have DTs?

Why was she hallucinating?

How do you treat overdoses of acetylsalicylic acid (aspirin)?

DISCUSSION Although this patient is indeed an alcoholic, she probably was not hallucinating due to alcohol withdrawal. She clearly does not have DTs; she is neither delirious nor tremulous. Scopolamine is a hallucinogen. In the past it was available in over-the-counter sedatives, but now requires a prescription. Other drugs such as bromides, lysergic acid (LSD), mescaline, and psilocybin may also cause hallucinations.

This patient's thirst, dry mouth, tachycardia, and dilated pupils are characteristic of an anticholinergic toxidrome. Some of the more common responsible drugs include scopolamine, tricyclic antidepressants, and antihistamines. This patient also had an anion-gap metabolic acidosis. Normally the anion gap (Na^+ + K^+ − Cl^- − HCO_3^-) is 8 ± 4 mEq/L. This patient was acidotic (HCO_3 9) with an anion gap of 28.8 mEq/L. We use the mnemonic *A MUD PILES* to remind us of the differential diagnosis of metabolic acidosis with an elevated anion gap.

A Alcohol

M Methanol
U Uremia
D Diabetic ketoacidosis

P Paraldehyde
I Iron/INH
L Lactic acid
E Ethylene glycol
S Salicylates

Salicylate toxicity is often underestimated since the patient is usually awake and alert. The serum salicylate level decreases over time as it is metabolized, so one should always check the "Done Nomogram" (a graphic representation of how fast the serum level drops) to see if the patient's serum level is in the toxic range for an ingestion hours earlier. If we do treat, it usually is with forced alkaline diuresis. We use a solution of 1000 ml 5% dextrose/0.45 normal saline plus 88 mEq $NaHCO_3$ plus 10 mEq KCl, and infuse it at 1000 ml per hour for the first hour. After the patient is fully hydrated, we use the same solution to keep urine output at around 3 to 6 ml/kg per hour (approximately 200 to 300 ml per hour in a normal-sized adult). This can produce pulmonary edema, so the patient must be watched carefully with chest x-rays, intake and output records, and chest auscultation. Since this can derange sodium or potassium levels and can produce dangerous levels of alkalosis, these parameters must be carefully monitored. Most of these patients need admission, especially if the salicylate level is over 80 mg per 100 milliliters.

In the end, alcoholism will be the patient's major problem; however, correction of her present metabolic abnormalities must precede any significant psychiatric therapy. She should not be obliged to admit to being an alcoholic to get such therapy. Alcoholism does not limit the patient's susceptibility to other drugs or diseases, but it often leads the physician away from a careful consideration of other diagnoses.

REFERENCES

Textbook   Rosen. Pp. 2141–2149.

Review Article   Riggs, B. S., Kulig, K., and Rumack, B. H. Current status of aspirin and acetaminophen intoxication. *Pediat. Ann.* 1987;16:888–898.

Additional   Snodgrass, W. R. Salicylate toxicity. *Pediatr. Clin. North Am.*
References   1986;33:381–391.

Hillman, R. J., and Prescott, L. F. Treatment of salicylate poisoning with repeated oral charcoal. *Br. Med. J.* 1985;291:1472.

Case 48 OD

A 45-year-old man was brought to the emergency department by ambulance. He was said to have ingested several drugs. On arrival he was drowsy but arousable. Although he refused to communicate, he could walk and had a good gag reflex. He was given syrup of ipecac, 30 ml orally, and 300 ml of warm tap water. This resulted in copious vomiting over the next thirty minutes. The patient was kept in the ED and observed. After three hours he seemed more alert and was walking about and asking the staff for cigarettes. He was referred to the emergency psychiatry team for further evaluation. Perusal of his old chart revealed that he had long carried the diagnosis of paranoid schizophrenia and had been on phenothiazines in the past.

The nurse on the psychiatry team saw the patient in the fifth hour of his ED stay and reported to the referring physician that he was too sleepy to interview. On rechecking he was found to be comatose and unresponsive to pain but breathing well and with a normal blood pressure. His pockets were emptied and found to contain prescription bottles for Thorazine, Seconal, and Kemadrin. A nasotracheal tube was easily placed, his stomach was lavaged with 2 liters of tap water via an Ewald tube, and he was admitted to the medical intensive care unit.

Why do overdose patients have fluctuating levels of consciousness?

What is "observation" in the ED?

DISCUSSION   The patient probably took more of his drugs covertly after entering the ED. He was a "double overdose." We occasionally observe an alcoholic becoming more drunk during his stay in the ED (more ataxic, sleepier, thicker speech) and find a half-full bottle of wine in his clothing. Usually overdose patients are stripped and searched and thus relieved of any drugs.

Varying depth of coma may be due to:

1. On and off gastrointestinal absorption. This is true for any drug but classic for meprobamate, which forms concretions in the gut. Duodenal storage may have been the problem here, and a cathartic should have been given.
2. Enterohepatic circulation.
3. Secondary effect of hypoxia on consciousness.
4. Brief action of narcotic antagonists versus long action of opiates.
5. Brief action of glucose versus long-acting hypoglycemic agents.
6. Subdural hematomas (especially worrisome in an alcoholic who is not properly waking up).
7. Repeated ingestion, as in this case.

This patient ingested three drugs with multiple side effects. They are all sedative-hypnotic drugs and may produce a decreasing level of consciousness and respiratory depression. Thorazine and Kemadrin (a drug used to treat extrapyramidal side effects of Thorazine) possess anticholinergic properties, and the patient should be monitored for cardiac arrhythmias, hypotension, seizures, and agitation.

Certain words have awesome implications in our ED that are not conveyed by their literal meaning. *Observed* should mean closely watched, yet often it is used to mean patient neglected, booth curtain closed, and no further evaluation. *Stable* is another such term. It should mean at least two successive observations the same with time intervening. It should not be used when we mean one set of normal vital signs with no temporal observations at all.

REFERENCES
Textbook   Tintinalli. Pp. 683–688, 692–693.

Review Article   Guzzardi, L. Phenothiazines and the Anti-psychotic Agents. In L. M. Hadadd and J. F. Winchester (eds.), *Clinical Manage-*

ment of Poisoning and Drug Overdose. Philadelphia, Saunders, 1983. Pp. 487–496.

Additional   Cann, H. M., and Verhulst, H. L. Accidental ingestion and over-
References   dosage involving psychopharmacologic drugs. *N. Engl. J. Med.* 1960;263:719–724.

Davis, J. M., et al. Overdosage of psychotropic drugs: A review. *Dis. Nerv. Sys.* 1968;29:157–164.

Case 49 Walking Away From a Car Accident

A 20-year-old man walked into the emergency department. He told the interviewing nurse that he had been in an auto accident three hours earlier but had felt more or less all right and had gone home. Then his shoulders, arms, and neck began to hurt, so his mother told him to go to the hospital. When he arrived, he was placed in an exam room, where he was interviewed by one of the more junior physicians available.

A full examination was done, including full range of movement of the neck. Then a complete set of cervical spine films was obtained, including flexion, extension, and odontoid views. The radiologist was not available, so the physician viewed the films alone. He mentioned to a staff physician that he had an interesting case of cervical spondylolisthesis. The second physician immediately placed sandbags on either side of the patient's head and a cervical collar on his neck. He told the patient not to move his head. A review of the films indeed disclosed an unstable cervical fracture-dislocation of C5-6. Skull tongs were placed, and the patient was admitted to the hospital for constant traction.

What is the usual presentation of a broken neck?

Is there anything unusual about this case?

What is the danger to the patient of further neck movement?

DISCUSSION   This patient had no apparent neurologic defect. By amazing luck his injury had not yet impinged on his cervical cord or nerve roots. The most common spinal fracture site is at the C6-7 vertebral level. A patient with that injury is brought in by stretcher with his arms flexed at the elbow and his hands together on his chest. He has flaccid paralysis elsewhere and may have hypotension due to loss of sympathetic innervation. It is not actually rare, however, for a patient with a cervical fracture to walk into our department unassisted and neurologically intact.

Accident victims brought in by ambulance should always be fully immobilized. This includes a hard cervical collar around the neck, sand bags on either side of the neck, and the patient strapped to a long spine board. Some patients will be immobilized this way even though they have no spine injury. In our ED, a patient that has *no* neck pain, has a normal mental status (not psychotic, somnolent, overly anxious, or under the influence of alcohol or drugs), and who has no neck tenderness on palpation or pain on gentle, slow, self-applied movement of the neck can have the neck "clinically cleared." All others must have their cervical spine x-rayed. Patients who present without full immobilization should be immobilized when they are first seen in the ED.

One should sandbag the patient's head straight. If it is turned, we usually try to straighten it *gently* with traction. If he is alert, he must be told to hold his head perfectly still, and if not, someone must constantly hold his head in place. This patient cannot be left alone. A cross-table lateral x-ray of the cervical spine should be done first. His arms should be pulled slowly down toward his feet before the x-ray—otherwise spasm of the shoulders may obscure much of the film below C5. Seven full cervical vertebrae must be seen for the film to be technically adequate. The x-ray should be carefully inspected for misalignment of the anterior and posterior border of the vertebral bodies and the anterior border of the spinous processes. The soft tissues anterior to the vertebral bodies should be examined for widening and the area of the odontoid (C2) closely looked at. The vertebral bodies themselves should be intact. If a fracture seems present, only an A-P film should then be taken and the patient immobilized by skeletal traction on the same stretcher with only one more move of the patient whenever possible— onto a circle bed or frame. If no fracture is seen on the lateral view, a full cervical spine x-ray series is obtained. In our institution this consists of A-P, odontoid view, and right and left oblique films. Flexion and extension views are occasionally used to evaluate the degree of ligamentous laxity but can be dangerous and should always be done under the guidance of an experienced physician.

Any movement may render the patient paraplegic or quadraplegic (depending on the injury level). If quadraplegia develops and is still present after twenty-four hours of traction, there is little chance of full recovery.

The three common types of incomplete cord injuries are:

1. Central cord syndrome—the patient may have weakness or flaccid paralysis of his arms and fairly normal legs. Note that this is the opposite of what one would usually expect with a spinal injury. The prognosis is usually good, and recovery usually takes place within hours.
2. Anterior spinal cord injury—loss of all but position and vibratory senses. The injury occurs (as do most spine injuries) with the neck flexed. Probably the anterior spinal artery is damaged. These cases may recover well if incomplete injury occurs.
3. Brown-Séquard syndrome—hemisection of the cord usually caused by a knife wound. There is a loss of position and vibratory sense on the side of the injury with loss of pain and temperature sense on the other side.

Incomplete cord syndromes may also present as combinations of all three types. Look for sparing of light touch sensation around the anus (sacral sparing) as a sign of incomplete damage. These cases have a better prognosis than a complete spinal cord transection.

A 1990 report by the National Acute Spinal Cord Injury Study demonstrated that methylprednisolone is surprisingly effective in treating both complete and incomplete spinal cord injury. If the drug was given in high dose and within 8 hours of the injury, significant improvement (motor and sensory) was seen in acutely injured patients.

REFERENCES

Textbook   Rosen. Pp. 419–471.

Review Article   Soderstrom, E. A., and Brumback, R. J. Early care of the patient with cervical spine injury. *Orthop. Clin. North Am.* 1986;17:3–13.

Additional References

Baker, J. S. The awake, alert patient can deceive (letter). *JACEP* 1978;7:289.

Harris, J. H., Edeiken-Monroe, B., and Kopanik, B. R. A practical classification of acute cervical spine injuries. *Orthop. Clin. North Am.* 1986;17:15–30.

Freemyer, B., et al. Comparison of five-view and three-view cervical spine series in the evaluation of patients with cervical trauma. *Ann. Emerg. Med.* 1989;18:818–821.

Macdonald, R. L., et al. Diagnosis of cervical spine injury in motor vehicle crash victims: How many x-rays are enough? *J. Trauma* 1990;30:392–397.

Bracken, M. B., et al. A randomized, controlled trial of methylprednisolone or naloxone in the treatment of acute spinal-cord injury. *N. Engl. J. Med.* 1990; 322:1405–1411.

Case 50 Hand Laceration

An 18-year-old man came to the emergency department after lacerating his left palm. He stated the accident occurred when he "broke a glass" while washing dishes. He was alert, well-mannered, and denied any other complaint. Though the ED was busy at the time he arrived, the patient's wound was bleeding briskly so he was quickly brought to a treatment booth. The physician, who was attending several other patients at this time, was summoned to see the patient. He quickly examined the wound and had the patient "make a fist," which he could easily do. The sensory exam was normal as well. The laceration was 2 cm in length, transversely placed just proximal to the fourth and fifth metacarpal phalangeal joints. The physician probed the wound and found no glass or bleeding arterial vessels. At this point, he anesthetized the wound with 5 ml of 2% plain Xylocaine solution and closed it with six 4-0 synthetic, nonabsorbable sutures. The wound was covered with an antimicrobial ointment, and a bulky dressing was applied. Prior to discharge the patient was given a diphtheria/tetanus toxoid booster since his last "tetanus shot" was over ten years previously. He was instructed to return for suture removal in ten days and subsequently discharged. Five days later he returned to the ED because of increasing pain in the area of the wound and because he noticed the wound had become red and tender. An x-ray of the hand was ordered at this time that revealed a 5 x 5 mm foreign body present deep in the soft tissues. Careful examination of tendon function revealed extreme pain on even 1 cm of passive motion of the fifth and fourth digits, as well as a diminished ability to flex the fourth finger at the distal interphalangeal (DIP) joint.

What are the complications from the initial injury that this patient is experiencing?

Was his initial treatment appropriate?

What should be done at this point?

DISCUSSION   Patients with hand lacerations involving the palm must be carefully examined. Unfortunately, it is very easy to miss a partial flexor tendon injury unless each superficialis and each profundus flexor tendon is examined! The profundus tendons each attach on the palmar surface of the digit's distal phalanx and are tested by asking the patient to bend the DIP joint with the rest of the finger immobilized. The superficialis tendons each insert on the flexor portion of the digit's middle phalanx and are tested by immobilizing the entire hand palm up on a flat surface, with only the finger in question free to move. If the patient can bend at the proximal interphalangeal joint, that flexor superficialis tendon is intact.

In this case, an injury to the profundus component of the flexor tendon was missed on the initial exam. Whenever there is a laceration in the soft tissues involving an object made of glass, particularly when that object shatters, suspicion must be high that a retained foreign body is present in the wound. Careful examination and exploration of the wound may not always reveal the foreign body. We do not know the true incidence of unsuspected retained glass fragments, but we sometimes recommend obtaining a "soft tissue density" x-ray in these situations since 95% of commercial glass is radiopaque.

On return, the patient also had evidence of wound infection that had extended into the flexor tendon sheath, a so-called flexor tenosynovitis. This is a dreaded complication of any penetrating wound to the palm area because permanently disabling adhesions may develop. The initial treatment of this particular patient should have included a careful flexor tendon exam. Had the foreign body and the flexor tendon injury been discovered on the initial visit, an appropriate consultation with a hand surgeon could have been obtained at that time and the complications might well have been avoided. In general, it is always a good idea to copiously irrigate such a wound using strict sterile technique.

This patient will now require hospitalization and intravenous antibiotics as well as surgical intervention to remove the foreign body. Whether or not the tendon sheath will require incision and drainage will be determined by response to antibiotic therapy.

REFERENCES

Textbook   Schwartz. Pp. 1422–1441.

Review Article   Lampe, E. W., and Netter, F. Surgical anatomy of the hand.
                      Ciba Clin. Symp. 1969;21:1–46.

Additional   Altman, R. S., et al. Initial management of hand injuries in the
References   emergency patient. *Am. J. Emerg. Med.* 1987;5:400–404.

                      Parry, R. O. *Acute Hand Injuries.* Boston, Little Brown, 1980.

Case 51 The Weekend Toothache

A 26-year-old woman walked into the emergency department complaining of severe pain in the site where one of her teeth had been removed four days previously. She said her dentist had warned her she might have some difficulty with unresolved infection and advised her to see an oral surgeon if any problems arose. He had then left town for the weekend. She was taking one acetaminophen with codeine every four hours for pain and 250 mg of penicillin every six hours.

She appeared to be in pain. Her vital signs included a pulse of 72, respiratory rate of 18, blood pressure of 140/90, and oral temperature of 99°F. Her mouth opened easily to reveal silk sutures in the empty socket with underlying clot, edema, and tenderness. No sign of gingivitis was seen around the other teeth. The gingival-buccal sulcus was unremarkable to inspection and palpation. The right maxillary sinus was tender to percussion. Sinus x-rays were obtained and showed mucosal thickening but no air-fluid level or opacification. The emergency physician changed her antibiotic to cefaclor and her pain medication to oxycodone and referred her to an otorhinolaryngologist the same day with a diagnosis of early maxillary sinusitis.

Two days later she returned to the ED saying she was in worse pain than before. Her vital signs were the same and her examination was the same except for increased tenderness. An oral surgeon was called in. He removed the sutures, probed the socket with a clamp, and released several milliliters of pus causing immediate improvement of the patient's pain.

What are the appropriate pain medications and antibiotics for dental infection?

What are common pathways of extension of dental infection?

When is it appropriate for the emergency physician to incise and drain a dental infection?

DISCUSSION   Oral and pharyngeal infections are appropriately treated with penicillin or a second-generation cephalosporin. Erythromycin is used in penicillin-sensitive individuals. Tetracycline is recommended for peridontal abscesses.

Both the dentist and the emergency physician used appropriate medications. The two problems in this case were insufficient surgical drainage of the infection and insufficient referral instructions.

Mandibular dental infection may spread through the soft tissue of the lower face and neck. Maxillary dental infection tends to spread through the upper half of the face and into the maxillary sinus. Advanced infections, especially in compromised hosts, may extend into any of the fascial planes of the neck and to the mediastinum.

If this patient's dentist had given her the specific name and phone number of an oral surgeon, she could have saved money and two days of pain by seeing him or her directly. The original emergency physician could have done her a similar favor by referring her directly to an oral surgeon the same day or by removing the sutures, or both.

If her abscess had presented with fluctuance in the gingiva facing the buccal mucosa or in the gingival-buccal sulcus, the emergency physician could have anesthetized the gingiva superficially with 2% lidocaine with epinephrine (1 : 100,000), incised the fluctuant area until pus was obtained, probed with a mosquito clamp, irrigated, and packed the abscess cavity with a small amount of iodoform gauze.

REFERENCES
Textbook   Rosen. Pp. 1055–1067.

Review Article   Gibson, E. E., and Verono, A. A. Dentistry in the emergency department. *J. Emerg. Med.* 1987;5:35–44.

Additional   Medford, H. M. Temporary stabilization of avulsed or luxated
References   teeth. *Ann. Emerg. Med.* 1982;11:490–492.

Klausen, B., Helbo, N., and Dabelsten, E. A differential diagnostic approach to the symptomatology of acute dental pain. *Oral Surg.* 1985;59:297–301.

Case 52 "No Fracture"

An 80-year-old man was brought to the emergency department by ambulance. He had fallen in his boarding home and could no longer walk because of right hip pain. He was in good general health but almost totally blind, the result of macular degeneration. He took no medicines, did not smoke, and drank no alcohol. On initial examination no remarkable abnormalities were noted except for his very poor vision and slight pain on rotation of his hip. An x-ray of the hip was obtained by the emergency doctor who could not find a fracture. He called in an orthopedist who agreed with the physical findings and the x-ray interpretation. "No fracture," he said, "This man can go home."

Accordingly, the patient was discharged home: that is, the medical record was filled out, signed, and "Home" checked in the disposition column. When a nurse went to escort the patient out, however, she found that he could not stand. The patient insisted that he had excruciating pain. He also explained to her that he lived two floors up in a boarding home without an elevator and that he had to come down to the dining room for meals. "How," he wondered, "can I get up and down for meals if I can't stand up?" The original physician had gone home by then so the nurse went in search of his successor. The new physician was puzzled. Since the orthopedist had discharged the patient and since he could not go back to his boarding home, what was to be done? The emergency physician called the orthopedist and after much conversation and some argument managed to have the patient admitted to the inpatient service. The patient spent twelve hours in the ED, during which time he was not fed because no one thought of it and because he was officially discharged during the greater part of the time.

What might the pathology have been that caused this man's hip pain?

What does this orthopedist need to know?

175

DISCUSSION   Hip pain after falls may be severe and incapacitating even in the absence of a fracture. Additionally, fractures of the hip or pelvis are often hard to find and may easily escape detection until several days after the initial injury. It was not clear whether the films taken in this case included adequate views of the entire pelvis to rule out a small pelvic fracture. Sometimes a fracture may be found with the aid of a bone scan even if invisible on x-ray, although the bone scan may be negative until 48 hours after the injury.

This orthopedist probably suffers from a common confusion that he is caring for fractures rather than for people. Perhaps he finds comfort in his specialization and hopes it will shield him from the need to participate in the care of real people. In this example, he was unable to see the elderly man who could neither stand nor walk, who could not return to his boarding house, and who needed care even though the pathology was unclear. The orthopedist needs to understand that he, like other doctors, will care for people in distress, some of whom will have medical problems that he understands and some of whom will not. In any case he will need to make greater efforts to help them.

REFERENCES
Textbook   Tintinalli. Pp. 905–907.

Review Article   Gertzbein, S. D., and Chenoweth, D. R. Injuries of the pelvic ring. *Clin. Orthop.* 1977;128:202–207.

Additional References   Freed, H. A., and Sheilds, N. N. Most frequently overlooked radiographically apparent fractures in a teaching hospital emergency department. *Ann. Emerg. Med.* 1984;13:900–904.

Frank, J. Physical diagnosis and the doctor–patient relation (letter). *N. Engl. J. Med.* 1976;294:1464.

Platt, F. W., and McMath, J. C. Clinical hypocompetence: The interview. *Ann. Intern. Med.* 1979;91:898–902.

Case 53 A Shooter with Vomiting

A 26-year-old man came to the hospital because he was vomiting and had lost his appetite. He reported that his illness had begun about three weeks earlier when he noted malaise and anorexia with slight nausea. He was able to take only fluids. He had begun vomiting everything he ate two days previously. He had night sweats but no fever. He also admitted to having some diarrhea, and his urine was darker than usual.

On examination, his temperature was 99.5°F, pulse 120, blood pressure 122/86, and respirations 26. He was not icteric. His skin showed multiple scars along the path of his arm veins. When confronted with these, he admitted that he had been an intravenous drug user for many years and was still actively shooting about $150 of heroin daily. He also admitted that he frequently shared needles. Further examination showed shotty cervical lymphadenopathy, and liver enlargement and tenderness. There were no bruises or spider angiomata. He felt lightheaded when he sat up, and a pulse in the upright position was 136, with a blood pressure of 118/86.

Blood was sent for complete blood count, liver enzymes, coagulation studies, BUN, glucose, and electrolytes. Tests for hepatitis A antibodies and hepatitis B surface antigen were also done. The staff nurse drawing the blood took extra care to prevent accidental needlesticks. An intravenous line of lactated Ringer's solution was begun, and he was given 2 liters over the next hour.

Since he could not keep any oral fluids down, he was admitted for intravenous hydration. An immediate consult was placed to the infectious disease service.

What is the emergency department treatment of the patient with acute viral hepatitis?

What are universal precautions against contact with the acquired immunodeficiency syndrome virus?

DISCUSSION   This patient probably has hepatitis and probably has the long-incubation or serum hepatitis type. He is not clinically icteric but may still have an elevated serum bilirubin. Most observers cannot detect jaundice until the total bilirubin is over 2 mg per 100 milliliters. Nevertheless, the urine may contain enough conjugated bilirubin ("direct-reacting bilirubin") to display yellow foam if shaken or to produce a positive dipstick reaction to bilirubin.

Hepatitis when seen in our ED is usually of viral or toxic etiology. The virus may be short-incubation "infectious hepatitis" with an incubation period of two to six weeks and hepatitis A antibody present. It may be parenterally transmitted long-incubation (six to twenty-four weeks) "serum hepatitis" with hepatitis B antigen present throughout the course. Hepatitis may be due to mononucleosis, indicated by a positive Monospot test. Viral hepatitis usually presents with a prodrome of several weeks of malaise, anorexia, and miscellaneous functional-sounding symptoms. A rash or arthralgias may begin the illness.

Toxins producing hepatitis include many chemicals and drugs. Antituberculosis therapy, halothane anesthesia, and others have been incriminated. In our ED the most common hepatotoxin is ethyl alcohol. Alcoholic hepatitis seems to act as a bridge between fatty liver and cirrhosis.

We usually obtain a weight on any presumed hepatitis patient. Anorexia or vomiting severe enough to cause continual weight loss may lead to hospitalization. In this case the patient's symptoms were so severe that he became dehydrated. The signs of increased thirst, dry lips, and light-headedness all suggest dehydration. Orthostatic vital signs are useful to demonstrate the presence of significant fluid losses. In our ED, a pulse increase of twenty points on standing from a lying position is considered a significant orthostatic change. This requires intravenous hydration, and if the patient is still unable to keep down fluids, he must be hospitalized. We draw biochemical survey, CBC, prothrombin time, hepatitis screen, and bilirubin (direct and indirect); and we obtain a urinalysis or a chest x-ray if findings suggest these.

Close contacts of patients with hepatitis A should receive gamma globulin as soon as possible to lessen the severity of the disease if they contract it. Any patient with presumed hepatitis A should be reported to the state health department by filling out the appropriate form. Contacts of hepatitis B patients, on the other hand, have far less chance of contracting hepatitis by an oral route. Sexual partners and persons who have had contact with the patient's blood need to be tested and treated. They should be tested for the presence of hepatitis B antigen and antibody, and if they are absent they should be given the hepatitis B vaccine and hepatitis B immune globulin. Other forms of infectious hepatitis include non-A, non-B hepatitis, and concurrent infection with the delta virus. This type of hepatitis is especially fulminant with a high mortality. ED personnel should be immunized against hepatitis B infection.

Acquired immunodeficiency syndrome (AIDS) is also spread primarily by the sharing of contaminated needles and through sexual contact with an AIDS virus carrier. Universal precautions should be followed in all EDs. These include the use of gloves for all procedures involving the possible contact with a patient's blood, wearing goggles when a likelihood of splattering exists, such as during intubation or irrigation of wounds; and assuming that *every* patient can have an infectious disease transmissible in the blood or secretions. Needles should never be recapped, and all soiled sharps should be disposed of in puncture-proof containers kept near the bedside.

Human immunodeficiency virus (HIV) infection is a diagnosis that is usually not made in the ED. Patients will frequently come to be tested for the "AIDS virus." We refer them to a site where appropriate counseling is given before and after the test is performed. AIDS patients will also present to the ED not previously diagnosed but complaining of what turns out to be the initial serious presentation of their disease. Most commonly this is a Pneumocystis carinii pneumonia, a diarrheal illness, or oral thrush. Many of these patients will require hospitalization because of poor followup in the community. Because of recent animal studies, we have now begun offering immediate treatment with AZT to anyone who has just had a high risk exposure to the AIDS virus. Anyone who has potentially infectious contact with blood from an HIV-positive patient should be tested at that time and again three and six months later. Failure to seroconvert after six months suggests that the person exposed did not acquire the virus, which luckily is much less contagious than hepatitis B.

REFERENCES

Textbook   Rosen. Pp. 1433–1444.

Review Article   Ruben, R. H. Acquired immunodeficiency syndrome. *Sci. Am. Med.* October 1988;1–15.

Additional   Baker, J. L. What is the occupational risk of emergency care
References   providers from the human immunodeficiency virus? *Ann.
                     Emerg. Med.* 1988;17:700–703.

                     Trott, A. Hepatitis B exposure and the emergency physician:
                     Risk assessment and hepatitis vaccine update. *Am. J. Emerg.
                     Med.* 1987;5:54–59.

                     Sken, W. F. Acquired immuno deficiency syndrome and the
                     emergency physician. *Ann. Emerg. Med.* 1985;14:267–273.

                     Hughes, W. T. Pneumocystis carinii pneumonia *N. Engl. J.
                     Med.* 1987;317:1021–1023.

                     Iserson, K. V., et al. Hepatitis B and vaccination in emergency
                     physicians. *Am. J. Emerg. Med.* 1987;5:227–231.

Case 54 Woman with Abdominal Pain

A 20-year-old woman came to the emergency department complaining of abdominal pain. She had been well previously and two days earlier had noted the onset of bilateral abdominal pain, most severe in the right lower abdomen, accompanied by nausea and vomiting. She had had no bowel movements for the past two days. She had noted no fever or chills and specifically denied any recent venereal disease or vaginal discharge. She was having sexual contacts and was on birth control pills. There was no prior history of abdominal or pelvic disease, and she had not had an appendectomy. Her last menstrual period had terminated three days earlier.

On physical examination, the patient appeared healthy but would pull away from an examining hand. Her blood pressure was 140/80, pulse 100, respiration 18, and temperature 38.0°C orally. The findings were normal except for her abdomen and pelvis. The abdomen was slightly distended, and she guarded throughout, especially the lower quadrants. Bowel sounds were present and unremarkable. The cervix was very tender, as were the uterus and adnexa. Because of this tenderness, the adnexa could not be clearly palpated. A rectal examination demonstrated the tenderness to be largely anterior to the examining finger. The stool was brown and negative for occult blood.

What is the diagnosis?

How should the patient be treated?

What are the most common misdiagnoses made in a case such as this?

DISCUSSION   Acute pelvic inflammatory disease (PID) is a common cause of
lower abdominal pain in young, sexually active women. It af-
fects 1% of women annually. The tubal scarring resulting from
PID is a leading cause of infertility and is probably responsible
for the recent increase in the rate of ectopic pregnancies in the
United States. The most common agents that cause PID are
*Neisseria gonorrhoeae, Chlamydia trachomatis, Myocoplasma
hominis, Ureaplasma urealyticum,* and anaerobic organisms.
The relative frequencies of occurrence of these agents are difficult to determine as only *N. gonorrhoeae* and *Chlamydia* are
routinely cultured.

Lower abdominal pain is almost universally present in PID.
The onset of pain often follows a menstrual period, during
which time the asymptomatic cervical infection ascends into the
upper tract. Fever, guarding, and rebound tenderness are seen
with advanced cases involving peritoneal irritation. Vaginal discharge and mucopurulent discharge from the cervical os are
commonly encountered. Marked cervical motion tenderness, a
tender nonenlarged uterus, and adnexal pain without adnexal
mass are typical and often clinch the diagnosis. Cultures should
be obtained for gonorrhea and *Chlamydia* in every young,
sexually active woman in whom a pelvic exam is performed
even if PID is not suspected. This is primarily for public health
reasons and will identify women who are asymptomatic or have
mild cervicitis.

In this woman the other differential diagnostic considerations
include appendicitis, ectopic pregnancy, ruptured ovarian cyst,
and endometriosis. The evaluation of abdominal pain should
always include a pregnancy test to help differentiate PID from
ectopic pregnancy and septic or spontaneous abortion. Ectopic
pregnancy can be fatal and typically presents with pelvic pain
worse on one side than the other. A tender unilateral adnexal
mass may be found. In our department we consider an ectopic
pregnancy ruled out by a negative *serum* pregnancy test
(BHCG). Unfortunately, we have seen patients with ectopic
pregnancies who on presentation had a negative *urine* pregnancy test. Pelvic ultrasound is often done in cases of pelvic
pain, when the pregnancy test is positive, to look for an ectopic.
If no intrauterine pregnancy is seen on ultrasound in a patient
with a positive pregnancy test, the patient should be admitted
as a presumed or "rule out" ectopic pregnancy. Early appendicitis may present with vague lower abdominal pain, fever, and
leukocytosis mimicking PID. The progression of the symptoms,
however, is usually different since the pain of appendicitis will

localize in the right lower quadrant, whereas PID almost always remains bilateral. A ruptured ovarian cyst will also produce lateralizing lower abdominal pain and occasionally rebound tenderness. Fever and leukocytosis are typically absent in this condition. Laparoscopy is occasionally necessary to differentiate the two. Endometriosis may also cause pain and occasionally peritoneal signs that mimick PID. A history of recurrent pain at the time of menses or a prior history of endometriosis is helpful in making a diagnosis.

Treatment of PID varies somewhat between institutions. Because of tubal scarring and the possibility of infertility, some experts feel a nulliparous woman or a woman desiring a larger family should be hospitalized and intravenous therapy given. In our department, patients with first episodes of PID are admitted (to retain the patient's fertility) as are patients with fever, marked-rebound tenderness, and signs of systemic toxicity. Likewise, we admit patients who do not respond to outpatient regimens, patients whose compliance with therapy is in doubt, and those in whom other conditions cannot be ruled out.

Outpatient therapy with ceftriaxone (250 mg intramuscularly) plus a ten- to fourteen- day course of oral doxycycline 100 mg bid is recommended. In addition to antibiotics, discharged patients should be rechecked in three days and told to avoid sexual intercourse for seven days. Followup examination should always be done to ensure adequacy of treatment. Instructions should be given to the patient to return for fever, increased pain, or intolerance of the medications. The patient should receive HIV counseling and have a VDRL drawn to screen for incubating syphilis. In addition, all sexual partners should be treated.

REFERENCES

Textbook Tintinalli. Pp. 378–380.

Review Article Goodrich, J. T. Pelvic inflammatory disease: Considerations related to therapy. *Rev. Infect. Dis.* 1982;4(Suppl.):S778–S787.

Additional Reference Centers for Disease Control. 1989 sexually transmitted diseases guidelines. *M.M.W.R.* 1989;38(No. S-8):21–34.

Case 55 The Blue Bruise

A 56-year-old man came to the emergency department complaining of pain in his right thigh. He had bumped it getting out of a car two days earlier, and it was getting more painful and swollen. Because his regular physician was out of town, he came to the ED. He had suffered a myocardial infarction six months earlier and was still on coumarin anticoagulant for this.

On examination, a large blue bruise covering the anterior lower right thigh was observed. A sample was drawn to check prothrombin time, and the patient was sent for an x-ray of the thigh. The x-ray was normal. By the time the patient returned from the radiology department, the physician caring for him had finished his twelve-hour shift and signed his cases over to another physician. The second physician noted that the x-ray pictures were normal and discharged the patient. The patient, however, was unsatisfied and went to another ED, where he was hospitalized. We later noted the prothrombin time to be 45 seconds with a control of 11 seconds.

Was this an example of a physician's error, a patient's error, or a failure of the medical system?

How should the patient have been treated?

What instructions should patients be given when they are placed on anticoagulant therapy?

DISCUSSION   This patient was handled correctly initially, but there was a lapse in care in the change of physicians. Obviously, if a laboratory test is worth doing, the results should be obtained and acted on. Fairly frequently a patient is signed over to another physician at a shift change, and the new physician fails to review the course of events properly and take over management of the problems being presented.

One must wonder why this patient did not question the second physician about the prothrombin time. He obviously was unsatisfied, but he did not communicate his dissatisfaction to the physician. Was this primarily a failure on the patient's part, a failure of the lab to provide data rapidly enough, or the physician's failure? Probably all three. Nonetheless, the physician must be assumed to have the ultimate responsibility.

Proper therapy for this patient would include bed rest, withdrawal of the anticoagulant, and probably some vitamin K to allow synthesis of needed clotting factors by the liver. Vitamin K is fat soluble and needs bile salts for absorption. If there is any suggestion of obstructive liver disease (intrahepatic or extrahepatic), the vitamin K should be given parenterally. To avoid another hematoma, it is usually given intravenously rather than intramuscularly in a 5- to 10-mg dose. Oral therapy is often acceptable. "Rebound hypercoagulability," an often-stated danger, probably is not as hazardous as overanticoagulation. Because his prothrombin time was so high (more than three times control), he probably also should have been treated with fresh frozen plasma to reverse his anticoagulation status. This was an example of a potentially unstable patient being dealt with as a nonemergent problem (even though he could have bled seriously with no warning at all).

Therapeutic anticoagulation with drugs related to coumarin is usually monitored with the prothrombin time. The prothrombin time is usually kept between one-and-a-half and two times the control. In any case, bleeding while on coumarin must be recognized as a dangerous problem. The patient must know that he should discontinue use of the anticoagulant and see his physician. He should also know that many other drugs are dangerous when he is on coumarin and that over-the-counter preparations should not be taken without checking with his physician. Most important, he should remind his physician when seeing him that he is on an anticoagulant. Patients usually assume their physicians remember everything, a dangerous assumption.

Whether or not the patient is on anticoagulants, the evaluation of soft tissue trauma should include examination of the area of injury and the joints immediately above and below the injury. Marked point tenderness, a large hematoma, injury at a joint, and limitation of function are factors that prompt an x-ray. Older patients can have extensive hematomas from relatively minor trauma. The detection of an exceptionally large hematoma should be followed by a CBC, platelet count, prothrombin time, and partial thromboplastin time.

REFERENCES

Textbook   Rosen. Pp. 1654–1660.

Review Article   Wessler, S., and Gitel, S. N. Warfarin. *N. Engl. J. Med.* 1984;311:645–652.

Additional   King, R. B., and Bechtold, D. L. Warfarin-induced illiopsoas
References   hemorrhage with subsequent femoral nerve palsy. *Ann. Emerg. Med.* 1985;14:362–364.

Scott, P. J. W. Anticoagulant drugs in the elderly: The risks usually outweigh the benefits. *Br. Med. J.* 1988;297:1261–1263.

Lowe, G. D. O. Anticoagulant drugs in the elderly: Valuable in selected patients. *Br. Med. J.* 1988;297:1260.

Case 56 Mistaken Identity, Shot in the Head

A 28-year-old policeman was brought to the emergency department by ambulance. He had made a call on a residence to investigate a prowler complaint. After an initial inspection, he knocked on the house door. The occupant reached around the partly opened door and fired a revolver at the policeman. Once the deed was done, he looked at his victim and called for an ambulance.

On arrival at the ED the patient was alive. He had a pulse and obtainable blood pressure of 140/80. His respirations were spontaneous at a rate of 14. He had an entrance wound between the eyebrows and an exit wound posteriorly just to the right of the occiput. His pupils were midposition and reactive. He was comatose with no response to voice or painful stimuli.

An endotracheal tube was placed, and the patient was hyperventilated with an Ambu bag at a rate of 30 per minute. Two intravenous routes were started and a solution of 5% dextrose in water was run very slowly at a keep-open rate. He was given 50 gm of mannitol. In the operating room an anterior craniotomy was done. The damaged right frontal lobe was debrided, the frontal sinus lining was curetted, and the craniotomy was closed. A similar procedure was done posteriorly. Two weeks later the patient left the hospital with a left hemiparesis.

How predictable is the outcome of head injury?

What is the reason for the hyperventilation and mannitol?

DISCUSSION   The priorities in treating this kind of trauma begin with the
ABCs. An adequate airway with ventilation and oxygenation
must be secured. If midfacial trauma is present, nasotracheal
intubation is contraindicated because the tube may penetrate
the cribiform plate and enter the brain. Massive oropharyngeal
hemorrhage may preclude orotracheal intubation and cricothyroidotomy may be necessary. Tracheostomy takes too
long and is almost never indicated in the ED setting.

The results of head injuries are not always predictable. One
should not hesitate to treat patients with even disastrous-ap-
pearing injuries.

In general, an anteroposterior bullet course is more likely to
be benign than a side-to-side wound. Nonetheless, many bul-
lets take courses not defined by a straight line connecting entrance and exit wounds. A high-velocity bullet tends to take a
straighter course than a low-velocity missile. Computed tomography can identify the extent of injury and bullet path and is
always indicated if an attempt is going to be made to save the
patient.

Initial therapy includes attempts at decreasing secondary injury by avoiding brain edema. Specific treatments include keeping intravenous fluids at a minimum, elevating the head of the
patient's bed, and hyperventilation (which is probably the most
effective maneuver). There is a saying that every medical specialty is allowed one irrational use of steroids. Nevertheless,
steroids (which lower intracranial pressure in some settings) are
of no proven benefit in head trauma, and many centers have
discontinued their use in patients like this. Mannitol at a dose of
1 to 2 gm per kg lowers intracranial pressure, but its use is
somewhat controversial unless herniation is present. No human
efficacy studies exist regarding the use of mannitol in head
injury. Neurosurgical therapy must be prompt even though the
brain is partly decompressed by the bullet wound of the cranium.

REFERENCES
Textbook   Tintinalli. Pp. 829–839.

Review Article Dagi, T. F. Emergency management of missile injuries to the
brain: Resuscitation, triage, and preoperative stabilization.
Am. J. Emerg. Med. 1987;5(2):140–148.

Additional References

Ordog, G. J., Wasserberger, J., and Balasubramanium, S. Wound ballistics: Theory and practice. *Am. Emerg. Med.* 1984;13:1113–1122.

Cushing, H. A study of a series of wounds involving the brain and its enveloping structures. *Br. J. Surg.* 1918;5:558–684.

Mace, S. E. Cricothyrotomy. *J. Emerg. Med.* 1988;6:309–319.

Case 57 EMS Radio Call

One morning in the emergency department, the EMS radio was activated and the following conversation took place:

Paramedic: Be advised we're on the scene with a 68-year-old white male, approximate weight 180 pounds, who suddenly became dizzy and complained of testicular pain and passed out. We found him on the floor, semiconscious, extremely diaphoretic. He is on the following medications: Slow-K, Minipress, and Lozol. Patient has no known allergies. His vital signs are as follows: respirations 28, pulse 104, systolic blood pressure 50, palpated. The patient has a history of high blood pressure, no other significant history. At this time the patient has a waxing and waning level of consciousness. We have him in MAST pants pumped up to 50.* We have an IV of lactated Ringer's running wide open in his left arm. We are attempting a second IV. We have a nonrebreathing mask, O_2 15 liters.† His ECG shows a sinus tach, his lungs are clear. Be advised the patient is complaining of some abdominal pain radiating to his back . . . [At this point the physician interrupted the paramedic.]

Physician: Peter, what's your ETA here?

Paramedic: Eight to ten minutes.

Physician: All right, it sounds like he's blowing an aneurysm. Blow up the MAST pants all the way including the abdominal segment. We'll be ready for you. Thanks a lot.

Paramedic: Thank you very much. We'll be there in eight to ten.

The physician immediately contacted the surgical house staff, described the patient, and asked that an operating room be prepared. Several minutes later the paramedic returned to the radio.

*50 mm Hg.
†Oxygen at 15 liters per minute.

Paramedic: Be advised the patient is awake now [audible patient groaning and ambulance siren in the background] and complaining. We're coming down the avenue and we'll be there in about three minutes.

Physician: Did you get a blood pressure, Peter?

Paramedic: We're getting one as we speak. Stand by.

Physician: Standing by.

Paramedic: Be advised the blood pressure is now 82 palp and he's had a liter-and-a-half of lactated Ringer's.

Physician: How many lines do you have in him?

Paramedic: We have two 14s.*

Physician: Stand by . . . [a brief pause] . . . You're going to booth six.

Paramedic: Thank you, Doc.

The patient was wheeled into the booth and a blood pressure was immediately obtained at 100 by palpation. Blood was drawn for routine preoperative studies and for typing and cross-matching of 6 units of blood. The patient was taken to the operating room within five minutes of his arrival in the ED. At operation he had a large ruptured aneurysm and an abdomen full of blood. He was discharged home eight days later.

Does all this radio jargon help?

What is the usual presentation of a ruptured or leaking aortic aneurysm?

---

*Two 14-gauge intravenous catheters.

DISCUSSION   This patient presented with classic signs and symptoms of a ruptured abdominal aortic aneurysm. It was probably because of the paramedic's clear communications and the physician's ability to use his findings quickly that the man survived.

The radio serves as the link between the paramedic and the physician providing medical control. Since paramedics are an extension of the emergency physician, his eyes, ears, and hands in the field, their communications must be precise. At the same time, in order to avoid delays in getting the patient treated in a timely manner, the communications must be brief and to the point. Some jargon allows shortcuts to be taken on the radio. The paramedics are trained in the "prehospital approach" to the patient. This follows a standard medical model of history, primary survey, and secondary survey. The primary survey is airway, breathing, and circulation followed by level of consciousness and vital signs. The secondary survey is a quick head-to-toe physical assessment of the patient to look for abnormal physical findings or injuries. Paramedics are not trained to diagnose. They are trained to always give the information in the same manner. This limits their attempts to make medical judgements in the field without medical control. When the communications are good, as in this case, rapid prehospital care and sometimes even diagnosis can occur.

Class I shock will present without any easily observable signs. (This is also called occult shock. It should be suspected when a mechanism of injury for shock is present and can sometimes be diagnosed by demonstrating a mild, otherwise unexplained metabolic acidosis.) Class II shock shows only tachycardia, tachypnea, and a decrease in pulse pressure. These changes occur when the patient has lost approximately 20% of his circulating blood volume. Class III shock presents with hypotension, marked tachycardia, and cool skin. This patient was near class IV hemorrhage. He had shock with severe blood loss (over 2000 ml), hypotension, plus evidence of end-organ failure (in this case central nervous system hypoperfusion). This degree of acute blood loss is immediately life-threatening.

The acute onset of testicular pain can also be caused by kidney stones, testicular torsion, or incarcerated hernia. When this patient was initially resuscitated with the MAST suit and intravenous therapy, he also complained of abdominal and back pain. These are common symptoms of acute aneurysmal rupture.

In the older population, a leaking aneurysm must always be considered in the differential diagnosis of abdominal or low back pain. Abdominal examination may show a pulsatile abdominal mass in the epigastrium (the bifurcation of the aorta is at the level of the umbilicus). Cross-table lateral and KUB films of the abdomen may show the aneurysm if its wall is calcified; and if leaking, it is usually greater than 5 cm in diameter. Further workup may include an abdominal ultrasound or computed tomography scan if the diagnosis cannot be made in the ED. If time allows, an aortogram will help the vascular surgeon immensely.

REFERENCES

Textbook   Rosen. Pp. 1197–1206.

Review Article   Perler, B. A., and Vertic, J. F. Abdominal aortic aneurysm: Diagnosing and treating on time. *Geriatrics* 1985;40:73–80.

Additional   O'Keefe, K. P., and Skiendzielewski, J. J. Abdominal aortic an-
References   eurysm rupture presenting as testicular pain. *Ann. Emerg. Med.* 1989;18:1096–1098.

                      Nevitt, M. P., Ballard, D. J., and Hallett, J. W. Prognosis of abdominal aortic aneurysm: A population based study. *N. Engl. J. Med.* 1989;321:1009–1014.

                      Crawford, E. S., and Hess, K. R. Abdominal aortic aneurysm (editorial). *N. Engl. J. Med.* 1989;321:1040–1042.

                      Caroline, N.L. *Emergency Care in the Streets* (2nd ed.). Boston: Little, Brown, 1983.

Case 58 Chronic Schizophrenic on Drugs

A 48-year-old man was brought to the emergency department by police car. His wife had called the police because he seemed confused and disoriented. He had been sitting in the bathroom brandishing a butcher knife and worrying about someone "coming for him." A mental health hold was placed, and he was brought to the ED.

On initial evaluation the following vital signs were obtained: blood pressure 130/90, pulse 120, temperature 37.6°C (99.7°F). He was said to be "a chronic schizophrenic on drugs." A sheriff's deputy who knew him stated that he frequently stopped taking his prescribed drugs and then "became more crazy." A physical examination showed a thick green material coating his teeth. His chest was thought to be clear. The initial impression was acute schizophrenia.

A second examiner was then asked to see the patient. He noted that the patient's skin was very warm, and a repeat temperature was taken. Because the patient could not keep his mouth closed on the thermometer, a rectal temperature was obtained and it was 39.9°C. The patient was noted to be tachypneic with a respiratory rate of 36. A more careful chest exam now showed rales, bronchial breath sounds, and dullness over the left lower lung field. The patient appeared terrified and kept looking over his shoulder "for the five men who were after him to gun him down as they had shot his three friends last week." The police could be sure that such a mass murder had not taken place. Although this material was clearly delusional, he otherwise made sense and expressed his fears clearly.

A chest x-ray showed a left lower lobe pneumonia. Subsequent calls to the patient's wife revealed that he had been drinking heavily until three days earlier. The patient was admitted to the hospital and placed on high-dosage parenteral penicillin and sedation. He had a tumultuous early course, with delirium, and then slow partial clearing of his pneumonia. An effusion persisted, and eventually he required surgical decortication of the left lower lobe.

How can you differentiate an acute organic brain syndrome from schizophrenia?

What is the differential diagnosis in a "confused" patient?

DISCUSSION   In this patient the temperature was the secret, and the first reading taken was erroneous. One must feel the patient and judge the approximate temperature. If the estimate is not close to the recorded value, retake the temperature and be careful to exclude artifactual errors such as mouth breathing or surreptitious heating of the thermometer by the patient. In the ED it is repeatedly made clear that the key to appreciation of the presence of severe disease lies in accurately reading vital signs. As one of our experienced clinicians likes to say, "They're not called *vital signs* for nothing." This patient had an acute toxic delirium and needed admission for intensive medical therapy.

Acute encephalopathy—usually metabolic rather than due to a mass lesion—can mimic a functional psychotic state fairly closely. We have seen intoxications with alcohol, antihistamines, scopolamine, amphetamines, cocaine, lysergic acid (LSD), and other medical problems confused with functional psychosis. Hypoxia, hypotension, or hypoglycemia may present with features suggesting schizophrenia. Subarachnoid hemorrhage, meningitis, and encephalitis have been misconstrued as nonorganic psychosis. Steroid psychosis and collagen disease vasculitis may present in this way.

In general, the differential diagnosis of a "confused" patient includes three main groups: *confusion, dysphasia,* or *schizophrenia.*

The acute metabolic encephalopathy patient is confused and usually somewhat agitated. He may have hallucinations, but these are usually visual (as opposed to the usually auditory ones in schizophrenia). The presence of a flap or ataxia, as well as the loss of orientation or the inability to do simple calculations, argues for metabolic brain disease. Any abnormality of vital signs should lead to a search for metabolic or toxic causes of encephalopathy. Blood sugar, blood alcohol, arterial blood gas, and serum sodium analyses are appropriate in any confused patient. Paranoid ideation is common to any acute encephalopathy and in no way differentiates metabolic disorders from schizophrenia.

The presence of perseveration, gibberish speech, or anger with the frustration of expressive difficulties may reveal the presence of dysphasia. Often such a patient can pick the right information from a list even if he cannot spontaneously answer questions. The dysphasic or aphasic patient may be oriented, although it may not be initially apparent, and has no hallucinations or gross delusions. Other neurologic abnormalities may indicate the presence of an old or new cerebrovascular accident.

Infections presenting with an acute organic brain syndrome (encephalopathy) are immediately life-threatening illnesses. Meningitis, pneumonia, urosepsis, and intra-abdominal infections are commonly associated with this syndrome, especially in the elderly, the alcoholic, or the immunologically deficient patient. Pneumonia is usually caused by gram-positive organisms, but with increasing age and debility the number of gram-negative organisms and unusual organisms increases. Meningitis can be caused by *Neisseria meningitides, Listeria, Escherichia coli,* or *Streptococcus.* Urinary tract infections leading to sepsis are usually due to gram-negative rods such as *E. coli, Pseudomonas,* or enterococci. Anaerobes or mixed gram-negative infections are commonly the cause of intra-abdominal infections that lead to sepsis. Many of these patients are unable to give a good history, and specific clues to the location of the infection may be absent, especially in the elderly.

Other conditions that can present this way include hyponatremia, hypercalcemia, renal and hepatic failure, porphyria, and the postictal state. The *ATOMIC*[5] mnemonic will help you recall the differential diagnosis of the common causes of acute encephalopathy:

A   Alcohol
T   Trauma
O   Overdose
M   Metabolic (hyponatremia, hypoglycemia, hypercalcemia, hepatic failure, hypoxia)
I   Infection (meningitis/encephalitis, brain abscess, acute febrile illness)
C[5] CVA, Cancer, Convulsion, Carbon monoxide, Cold (hypothermia)

REFERENCES

Textbook   Rosen. Pp. 1103–1117, 2251–2257.

Review Article   Zun, L., and Howes, D. S. The mental status evaluation—Application in the emergency department. *Am. J. Emerg. Med.* 1988;6:165–172.

Additional   Zisook, S., and Baraff, D. L. Delirium: Recognition and man-
References   agement in the older patient. *Geriatrics* 1986;41:67–78.

Lipowski, Z. J. Delirium (acute confusional states). *J.A.M.A.* 1987;258:1789–1792.

Erkinjuntti, T., et al. Short portable mental questionnaire as a screening test for dementia and delirium among the elderly. *J. Am. Geriatr. Soc.* 1987;35:412–416.

Case 59 Acute Myocardial Infarction

A 50-year-old man was sent to the outpatient lab by his family doctor for some routine blood work to monitor his hypertension and mild diabetes. While the phlebotomist was drawing his blood, the patient became weak and felt a slight pressure in his chest. The laboratory technician called an orderly who found a wheeled stretcher and brought him to the emergency department. In the department he was placed on a cardiac monitor, oxygen by nasal prongs was administered, and an intravenous line of 5% dextrose in water was begun. The monitor showed obvious ST-segment elevation.

A twelve-lead ECG was immediately done. It showed ST-segment elevations and T-wave inversions in leads II, III, and aVF, with reciprocal changes in I and aVL. The ED attending physician decided to begin treatment with tissue plasminogen activator (TPA) to attempt to dissolve what she assumed to be a coronary thrombosis.

Four intravenous lines were begun and heparin and TPA infusions were started. The patient's chest discomfort was treated with two nitroglycerin tablets sublingually with complete relief. Within ten minutes of the onset of the infusion, the elevated ST segments on the monitor were no longer present, and the patient felt much better. He had a few runs of ventricular tachycardia of four and five beats each. Lidocaine was given by bolus and a constant infusion was begun. No further arrhythmias occurred. The patient was admitted to the coronary care unit as soon as a bed was available.

What is the standard treatment for an acute myocardial infarction?

When is TPA useful?

When should lidocaine be used prophylactically?

Can you diagnose an acute myocardial infarction from seeing ST-segment elevation on the cardiac monitor?

199

DISCUSSION   Two major problems face the emergency physician who deals
with patients with chest pain or other symptoms possibly due to
coronary artery disease.

The first problem is the task of identifying which patients are
likely to die suddenly. This is not entirely possible with available
methods and is not synonymous with identifying patients who
are suffering myocardial infarctions. Even the diagnosis of an
acute myocardial infarction is not always easy. Frequently the
patient does not present with a textbook description of crushing
central chest pain associated with weakness, nausea, and diaphoresis. The patient may suffer a myocardial infarction and yet
clearly deny chest pain. To approach this problem we suggest
the following steps:

1. The history is the best source of data. Above all, do not
   invest too much security in the ECG. A normal ECG in no
   way precludes sudden death.
2. If a history of pain is not forthcoming, listen more for the
   circumstances surrounding the patient's decision to call for
   help. What was he doing and how did he feel? A patient who
   denies much pain but says he felt that he was about to die
   probably should be admitted to the coronary care unit.
3. The physical examination must search for evidence of congestive heart failure, for an abdominal problem simulating
   myocardial ischemia, and for arrhythmias. The pulse should
   be carefully felt.

The next priority is that of preventing sudden death if possible. Any patient with chest pains that might conceivably be of
cardiac origin needs three things right away: an intravenous
line, oxygen, and a cardiac monitor. This should happen as
early in the workup as is practical. The monitor is helpful in
picking up arrhythmias but cannot diagnose an acute myocardial infarction since monitor ST-segment elevations may be artifactual. True ST-segment elevation is seen on a standard
twelve-lead ECG.

Patients who have acute myocardial ischemia are given nitroglycerin and morphine as needed for pain. This therapy will
also improve coronary blood flow and decrease myocardial
work and oxygen consumption. Since most cardiac arrests early
in a myocardial infarction are due to ventricular fibrillation, any
arrhythmia should be quickly diagnosed and treated. New, mul-
tifocal, or frequent premature ventricular contractions, couplets
(bigeminy or trigeminy), or runs of premature ventricular con-

tractions should be treated with lidocaine.

The next task is that of initiating treatment to limit the size of the infarction. Of the various therapies that have been tried for this, thrombolysis seems the most effective. If there is ST-segment elevation in contiguous leads and the patient has had pain for less than four hours, thrombolytic therapy should be started if possible. We use TPA to accomplish thrombus dissolution. Streptokinase and urokinase are also widely used. TPA is contraindicated in any patient who has a bleeding disorder, recent surgery, bleeding ulcer, stroke, or prolonged cardiopulmonary resuscitation. Heparin and intravenous nitroglycerin are given at the same time. Reperfusion arrhythmias are a common sign of clot dissolution. We usually treat these with lidocaine.

The patient needs rapid evaluation, rapid decision-making, and safe transportation from the ED to the coronary care unit. No time should be lost in the x-ray unit, and a physician with a portable monitor defibrillator should accompany the patient to the coronary care unit.

REFERENCES

Textbook   Tintinalli. Pp. 191–198.

Review Article   Walsh, D. G., et al. Use of tissue plasminogen activator in the emergency department for acute myocardial infarction. *Ann. Emerg. Med.* 1987;16:243–247.

Additional References   Braunwald, E., and the TIMI Study Group. Comparison of invasive and conservative strategies after treatment with intravenous tissue plasminogen activator in acute myocardial infarction: Results of the thrombolysis in myocardial infarction phase II trial. *N. Engl. J. Med.* 1989;320(10):618–627.

Bressler, M. J. Future roles of thrombolytic therapy in emergency medicine. *Ann. Emerg. Med.* 1989;18:1331–1338.

Kennedy, J. W., et al. Recent changes in management of acute myocardial infarction: Implications for emergency care physicians. *J. Am. Coll. Cardiol.* 1988;11:446–449.

Smith, M. Thrombolytic therapy for myocardial infarction: A pivotal role of emergency medicine. *Ann. Emerg. Med.* 1987; 16:592.

Case 60 Facial Trauma

A 48-year-old woman came to the emergency department claiming that she had been in a fight with her husband. She smelled of alcohol, was disheveled, and lapsed into tears periodically. She had multiple puffy, bruised areas about her face, and her nose was obviously crooked. Both eyes were puffy, and one was almost shut. She was breathing easily and had normal vital signs. The resident radiologist recommended sinus views and a nasal view. The only abnormality of the bones was a fractured nose. She was sent home with an ice pack and told to return the next day to the ear-nose-throat (ENT) clinic to have her nose adjusted.

How do you determine what is broken in facial trauma?

What x-ray views may be helpful?

What about sending this woman home?

DISCUSSION The first concerns in facial trauma have to do with airway, neck, and brain injuries. Laryngeal trauma can accompany facial trauma, and laryngeal edema may be progressive. Once these are dealt with, the bones of the face should be carefully palpated. Both sides must be compared at each step. Palpate the zygomatic arch, the orbital rim, the maxilla, and the jaw. Anesthesia of the infraorbital nerve suggests a fracture. The most important question to ask a patient with a suspected mandibular or maxillary fracture is whether her teeth fit together properly. The physical examination of the face should also include an examination of the nasal septum for signs of a septal hematoma and if present it should be evacuated. Visual acuity should be checked when there is any injury of or around the eyes. If the acuity is less then perfect, attempt correction by having the patient look through a pinhole or use her glasses. If the vision corrects, the problem is refractive only. If it does not correct, look for other results of eye trauma such as a hyphema, traumatic glaucoma, ruptured globe, or retinal detachment. A slit lamp examination is mandatory when there has been visual loss. If the extraocular movements are unequal or incomplete, suspect entrapment of one of the extraocular muscles in an orbital floor fracture.

Midface fractures may be maxillary—usually occurring in major trauma such as those sustained in auto accidents. They may be blowout fractures of the orbit with an intact orbital rim and orbital floor collapse. They may be tripod fractures of the zygomatic arch, or they may be nasal fractures. There may be cerebrospinal rhinorrhea and associated basal skull fractures. Of all these, the nasal fracture is most common and most benign. We usually do no emergency manipulation of a nasal fracture. We inspect the nasal septum for the presence of a septal hematoma and, if none is found, we just arrange for follow-up in 3–5 days.

Mandibular fractures may present with many loose foreign bodies (e.g., teeth) that can be aspirated by the patient if she is at all obtunded and lying on her back. There are often associated mouth wounds, making the fracture compound. In such cases we usually close all layers of the laceration and give the patient antibiotics. Ice packs should be applied to all facial contusions to decrease the swelling as rapidly as possible. The avulsed or loose teeth should be treated by a dentist or oral surgeon as soon as possible. Teeth may be reimplanted, but the success rate decreases rapidly as the time from the injury increases. If the tooth has fallen out of its socket, it should be rinsed off and replaced.

There are many possible x-rays for facial fractures. The best view is one that includes the bone that is fractured—the one with the greatest tenderness or swelling over it. Specific bones should be x-rayed rather than ordering a general facial series. An upright Waters' view of the maxillary sinuses will frequently show fluid in the maxillary sinuses or a blowout of the floor of the orbit. Special dental films are often necessary to demonstrate tooth fractures. Maxillary and mandibular fractures may be best seen on a Panorex view of the mouth, and special "jughandle" views show most clearly the zygomatic arches.

Finally, victims of violence should be offered counseling and referred to a safe place to stay. Most cities have battered women's shelters where women who have been victims of domestic violence can go to be safe from further attacks. Returning this woman home with no effort to deal with the violence is shortsighted. The facial injuries are trivial compared to the marital disorder and its potential for even more disastrous results. The patient may need protection. Her husband may need help too.

REFERENCES

Textbook   Rosen. Pp. 395–410.

Review Article   Shepherd, S. M., and Lippe, M. S. Maxillofacial trauma: Evaluation and management by the emergency physician. *Emerg. Med. Clin. North Am.* 1987;5:371–392.

Additional   Seton, J. R. Soft tissue facial injuries related to vehicular acci-
References   dents. *Clin. Plastic Surg.* 1975;2:79–92.

                        Baker, S. P., and Schultz, R. C. Recurrent problems in emergency room management of maxillofacial injuries. *Clin. Plast. Surg.* 1975;2:65–71.

Case 61 Laceration

A 30-year-old man was brought to the emergency department by ambulance after his family called the city emergency number 911, reported that he was bleeding seriously from a cut, and requested an ambulance. The policeman who arrived minutes before the ambulance found a husky man with a tourniquet on his left upper arm and a 4-cm wound laterally on his forearm. They replaced the tourniquet with a bath towel local-pressure bandage. The ambulance attendant removed this and found a no-longer-bleeding wound, which he bound with a sterile dressing.

Before leaving the scene, the ambulance attendant followed the trail of blood through the patient's house to the basement, where he noticed a small wooden table with a sharply broken leg. The table leg was splintered, and the attendant noted the possibility of splinters in the wound. He estimated there was about 500 ml of blood about the house.

On his arrival at the ED, the patient's wound was anesthetized, cleaned, and irrigated. A gloved finger could be inserted subcutaneously for about 8 centimeters.

How do lay persons generally try to stop bleeding?

How would you treat this wound?

DISCUSSION   It is amazing how few people realize that pressure over a wound is appropriate to hold bleeding in check. We have people appearing at the ED who have tried to stop bleeding by applying anything from vitamin A to turpentine to the wound. Most people seem to be of the "dab and look" school, applying inadequate pressure for inadequate time and then checking to see if it is still bleeding. This patient probably lost a unit of blood, thanks in part to a tourniquet applied at too low a pressure. Fortunately, his family called 911 to access professional prehospital care for his wound; without it, he could have bled to death. EMTs usually attempt to stop bleeding by direct pressure and the application of a pressure bandage. If that fails, pressure on the artery proximal to the wound is attempted in addition to direct pressure. Tourniquets are only applied as a last resort as a lifesaving measure when other less potentially damaging maneuvers fail. The time a tourniquet is applied should be well documented on the patient's medical record. As a safety measure, we always write the time applied on the patient's skin next to the tourniquet.

The keystone of wound care is adequate debridement. All wounds are contaminated. Problems that arise almost always can be traced to ineffective removal of this contamination during initial treatment. Wounds are contaminated by damaged or dead tissues and by ground-in dirt and bacteria. Removal of dead or damaged tissue and ground-in dirt or bacteria will leave a wound that heals primarily, leaving a minimal scar. Removal of dead or damaged tissue is accomplished by sharp excision of obvious necrotic material and ragged subcutaneous tissue, with "freshening up" of skin edges. This can be done with fine (Iris) scissors or a scalpel. Removal of embedded dirt or bacteria can be accomplished by copiously irrigating the depths of the wound with a 20-ml syringe and a 20-gauge needle (or similar narrow lumen device) using at least 500 ml of saline solution for a moderate laceration (5 to 6 cm) and more for a larger laceration. This cannot be adequately done in a wound that has not been adequately anesthetized.

This patient's wound was opened with a scalpel to the full extent of the undermined tunnel. Several splinters of wood were removed. The rough skin edges were debrided and the opened wound rescrubbed and irrigated. As with all deep lacerations, this wound was closed in layers. Subcutaneous tissue may consist of fat, muscle, and fascia, but since neither fat nor muscle holds sutures very well, we usually only sew fascial layers and the skin. Any buried (absorbable) suture material is acceptable, but we avoid both plain gut and "chromic" because they get sticky when wet and lack tensile strength. Many types and brands of skin (nonabsorbable) sutures are available, and it makes little difference which you use. Silk is popular since it is so strong and easy to use. Unfortunately, it is also quite inflammatory and tends to leave suture marks. Our common practice is to use 3–0 silk for scalp and intraoral wounds and 4–0 to 6–0 nylon or Prolene elsewhere. Tetanus prophylaxis for most clean wounds is given if it has been more than ten years since the last dose of tetanus toxoid. If no primary immunization has been given, or if it was inadequate, tetanus immunoglobin should be considered also. Sutured wounds are initially susceptible to infection by invasion from the outside, so after an initial cleaning in the ED we ask the patients to keep their wounds clean and dry for forty eight to seventy-two hours. Antibiotic prophylaxis for most wounds will not prevent a secondary infection and generally should not be used.

Sutures are removed in three to five days for facial wounds, seven to ten days on most average wounds, and ten to fourteen days on slow-to-heal areas such as the feet or over a joint. Because this patient's injury was deep and contaminated, he was told to return to the ED in two days to have his wound reexamined.

REFERENCES

Textbook   Schwartz. Pp. 465–475.

Review Article   Edlich, R. F., et al. Principles of emergency wound management. *Ann. Emerg. Med.* 1988;17:1284–1302.

Additional References   Lammers, R. L. Soft tissue foreign bodies. *Ann. Emerg. Med.* 1988;17:1336–1347.

Christoph, R. A., et al. Pain reduction and local anesthetic administration through pH buffering. *Ann. Emerg. Med.* 1988; 17:117–120.

Zitelli, J. A. Maximizing a wound's potential for healing. *Emerg. Med. Rep.* 1989;10:83–92.

Bartfield, J.M., et al. Buffered versus plain lidocaine as a local anesthetic for simple laceration repair. *Ann. Emerg. Med.* 1990;19:1387–1389.

Case **62** Constipation

A 77-year-old woman was brought to the emergency department complaining of constipation. She had had trouble with bowel function for over ten years and had been diagnosed as having Parkinson's disease for the past five years. At present she was on L-dopa and 1 teaspoonful of Metamucil daily. She complained of diffuse abdominal cramping pain, vomiting, and squirts of diarrhea despite a feeling of inability to pass a stool. On physical examination she had normal vital signs and a mildly tender abdomen. Her rectum was vastly distended by soft, brown stool that tested negative for occult blood.

The physician caring for her thought that she had obstipation resulting in a partial rectal obstruction.

Does Parkinson's disease lead to constipation?

How should the patient be treated?

When is constipation a sign of more serious disease?

DISCUSSION   Most patients with Parkinson's syndrome are old, and colonic malfunction is common in the old. Probably the neurologic disease itself does not lead to constipation, but of course, such patients are often treated with anticholinergics, and these drugs may induce more bowel dysfunction.

Therapy should begin with vigorous cleaning out of the distended rectum. This can usually be done with enemas. After they were unsuccessful in this patient, she was given 10 mg of morphine subcutaneously. Nupercaine anesthetic ointment was placed in the anal canal, and the impaction was removed bit by bit digitally.

The woman was then allowed to rest for an hour and sent home with instructions to use a tap water enema once a day for three days; to drink at least 2 quarts of fluid daily; to take 2 teaspoonfuls of Metamucil in water qid followed each time by a glass of hot water. She was encouraged to take a large glass of prune juice each morning; not to ignore any urge for a bowel movement; to increase her intake of fiber and fluids; and to set aside a time each morning after breakfast to attempt a bowel movement. She was told that if she went three days with no evacuation she should use glycerine suppositories, and, if that was unsuccessful, a tap water enema.

Since the diarrhea is a sort of overflow incontinence as a result of obstipation, opiates would be antitherapeutic and should not be used.

Of course people mean all sorts of different things when they cite "constipation," and the physician's first task is to translate the code. Then, at the very least, abdominal and rectal exams are needed to make sense of the problem.

One good way to stay out of trouble in the practice of emergency medicine is for the physician to consider in each case what is the worst thing that could be accounting for the patient's current symptoms. Constipation may be a local problem involving rectal dysfunction, as in this case, or it can be a sign of severe underlying disease. Particularly in the elderly patient, it can be difficult to differentiate between simple constipation and the low-grade ileus that often is seen as the first sign of an impending bowel obstruction or acute abdomen.

REFERENCES
Textbook   Rosen. Pp. 1514–1515.

Review Article   Wrenn, K. Fecal impaction. *N. Engl. J. Med.* 1989;321:658–
                        662.

Additional   Tedesco, F.J., and DiPiro, J.T. Laxative use in constipation. *Am.*
Reference   *J. Gastroenterol.* 1985;80:303.

Case 63 Difficulty Swallowing

A 66-year-old woman presented to the triage nurse stating that she had eaten some chicken a day before and swallowed a bone. She thought that it was stuck in her throat. When asked where she felt it, she pointed at her mid neck. She said she could swallow, but then regurgitated everything including her saliva. She was comfortable and able to speak normally and had normal vital signs. Initial examination disclosed discomfort on laryngeal palpation but no other abnormalities. Because of the localization of her symptoms, a soft tissue x-ray of the neck was ordered. This showed what appeared to be a chicken bone sticking out of the upper esophagus. After her palate and posterior larynx were anesthetized with Cetacaine spray, indirect laryngoscopy was performed using a lamp, a head mirror, and a heated dental mirror. No foreign body was seen. After the patient was successfully able to take a sip of water, she was discharged.

Before she left, however, a more senior resident working in the department called her back. He sent her back to x-ray for a barium swallow that revealed a filling defect in the esophagus at the gastroesophageal junction. She was promptly sent to the gastrointestinal lab for esophagogastroscopy.

What constitutes a choking emergency?

How is a choking emergency treated?

What is the treatment of a nonemergent gastrointestinal foreign body?

DISCUSSION   Esophageal obstruction commonly presents in this way, and
meat impaction is common even without the presence of organic disease of the distal esophagus. There is much discomfort
and a serious potential for emesis with aspiration. The patient
should be taken seriously and treated quickly. If the patient is
seen after about one hour, she is usually drooling copious
quantities of saliva. She often sits quietly with her head bowed
over a towel or basin and can be diagnosed from across the
room. Barium swallow is a valuable diagnostic tool, but you
must be careful that the patient does not aspirate any barium.

We do not advise the use of enzymes or meat tenderizer;
these agents are very irritating and destructive to an already
damaged esophageal mucosa. One or two milligrams of glucagon given intravenously may result in passage of the foreign
body. If not, the patient needs endoscopy, which is usually done
with local anesthesia after sedation.

Most foreign bodies, even sharp objects, that pass into the
stomach will pass harmlessly through the intestines. Though
there is debate about the safety of waiting for the passage of a
sharp object, we believe that for the reliable patient, invasive
action is required only when pain or obstruction develops.

A "café coronary" refers to the sudden death of a restaurant
patron choking on a large piece of food. This is usually steak
and the patient usually has consumed several alcoholic bever-
ages. The patient may have dentures or may be a loud talker
while eating. The food lodges in the hypopharynx and pushes
the trachea closed or obstructs in the glottis. Treatment must be
immediate or all is lost. Café coronary patients do not make it
to the ED. The Heimlich maneuver is lifesaving in these patients. It consists of standing behind the patient and placing both
arms around her with your hands making one fist on the upper
epigastrium just below the xiphoid. Pressure is exerted with a
quick upward and inward movement of the fists. This should
expel the obstructing mass. If four thrusts are unsuccessful, try
to remove the food with a finger sweep of the posterior hypopharynx being careful not to ram the bolus deeper. (If the
equipment is available, use Magill forceps.) If none of this clears
the airway, a stab wound cricothyroidotomy should be done.
Despite the name, the coronary arteries are not implicated in
this illness.

In this patient the "chicken bone" that was seen on x-ray of
the neck was later reread by the radiologist as a calcified hyoid
cartilage. The patient was taken to the operating room where a
large bolus of meat was pushed out of her esophagus and into

the stomach by an endoscope.

REFERENCES

Textbook   Tintinalli. Pp. 301–306.

Review Article   Hernanz-Schulman, M., and Niemark, A. Avoiding disaster with
                      esophageal foreign bodies. *Emerg. Med. Rep.* 1984;special
                      issue:133–140.

Additional   Nandi, P. E., and Ong, G. B. Foreign body in the oesophagus:
Reference   Review of 2,394 cases. *Br. J. Surg.* 1978;65:5.

Case 64 Allergic to Shrimp

The fire department paramedics were called to a local restaurant. They went to the scene where a 43-year-old woman was complaining of having an allergic reaction. She stated that she was allergic to shellfish and that she had accidently eaten a salad containing some shrimp. She realized her error too late.

In minutes she began itching and was now covered with hives. She also complained of having some difficulty breathing. The paramedics reported that her skin was indeed covered with hives but her lungs were clear. Her pulse was 110 and her blood pressure was 100/60. Her respiratory rate was 28 and slightly labored. The paramedics started a rapid intravenous infusion of lactated Ringer's solution and contacted the medical control physician by radio for further orders. The medical control physician on duty ordered epinephrine 0.3 mg to be given subcutaneously. The MAST garment was to be applied but not inflated unless the patient's blood pressure went below 100 systolic. The paramedics' estimated time of arrival at the emergency department was ten minutes.

When the patient arrived in the ED, she felt somewhat better. Her vital signs had not changed. She was given diphenhydramine and methylprednisolone intravenously and admitted to the hospital for an observation period.

What kinds of allergens predispose to anaphylaxis?

What are the priorities in the treatment of anaphylaxis?

How can paramedics treat complex medical emergencies in the street?

DISCUSSION Anaphylaxis occurs immediately after reexposure to an allergen. Common allergens causing anaphylaxis include penicillin, peanuts, fish, and insect venom. The antigen-antibody interaction usually causes hives, wheezing, laryngeal edema (hoarseness), and occasionally shock. Shock is a state in which vital organs are inadequately profused; anaphylactic shock is caused by decreasing the vascular tone and increasing vascular permeability.

In the early stages of the anaphylactic syndrome, the patients may complain of thirst, light-headedness, shortness of breath, gastrointestinal symptoms, a marked warmth and flushing of the skin, and pruritus (typically, intense itching of the palms of the hands). Laryngeal edema, marked wheezing, and hypotension develop later. Most patients with anaphylaxis respond to epinephrine, but some require endotracheal intubation or cricothyrotomy. The epinephrine is usually given subcutaneously for mild to moderate cases and intravenously or endotracheally for severe anaphylactic shock. Intravenous epinephrine has two undesirable features: a high peak blood pressure and a very short duration of action. We only use it in the most severe cases.

Patients with anaphylactic shock or laryngeal edema should be admitted for an observation period. Anaphylactoid reactions without shock or severe airway obstruction may be observed in the ED for a few hours and the patient then released on oral steroids and antihistamines.

Paramedics are allied health professionals trained to recognize and begin treatment of medical emergencies at the scene of the illness or injury. Some areas of the country allow paramedics to administer epinephrine on standing orders (previously agreed on protocols), but most require some sort of physician contact. This "on-line" medical control occurs when the paramedic establishes radio or phone communications with a physician, presents the patient's history and physical findings, and requests orders for further treatment. The use of crystalloid infusions by large intravenous lines is usually allowed under standing orders, but after they are begun the medic must contact the medical control authority for further orders. Some prehospital care systems allow the use of diphenhydramine or steroids. Anaphylaxis is one of the serious medical emergencies that can be nearly cured prior to the patient's arrival at the hospital.

REFERENCES
Textbook   Rosen. Pp. 203–225.

Review Article   Netzel, M. C. Anaphylaxis: Clinical presentation, immunologic
                        mechanisms, and treatment. *J. Emerg. Med.* 1986;4:227–
                        236.

Additional   American College of Emergency Physicians. Guidelines for
Reference   emergency medical services. *Ann. Emerg. Med.* 1988;17:
                        742–745.

Case 65 Pediatric Head Injury

A 2-year-old boy was brought to the emergency department by his concerned parents because he seemed unduly sleepy and had vomited several times. Three hours earlier he had fallen off the top bunk of a double bunk bed, landing on his right side and hitting the right side of his head.

On arrival in the ED, he seemed alert and would cry vigorously if stimulated. He could walk well and move all extremities well, had equal and reactive pupils, and had no facial or head abnormalities. He had no evidence of other injuries and had made no prior visits to the ED for injuries. A skull series of x-rays was done; they were unremarkable.

How unusual is it for children to vomit after head injuries?

Should a head computed tomogram be done?

Is this a case of a "battered child"?

What are the usual features of a case of child battering?

DISCUSSION   Although vomiting is a serious symptom in an adult with head injury, it is of less diagnostic significance in a child, since it is present in a high percentage of children with relatively trivial head injuries. This child, like all others with head injury, needs careful observation over the ensuing twenty-four hours. He should be watched for arousability and the development of gross focal neurologic defects. Since he has a responsible family, we will send him home with careful instructions. We tell the parents to wake him every two hours and have him touch the parent's finger tip and walk him to the bathroom. If he can do these highly coordinated maneuvers with ease, he has been adequately observed and can go back to bed for two more hours. An alarm clock must be set at two-hour intervals. Of course, if he deteriorates, he must be returned to the ED and studied further. If the parents are deemed unreliable, then the child must be admitted for observation.

Computed tomography (CT) has replaced all other modes to identify acute intracranial injury. A consensus on exact indications for CT in head trauma is still evolving. We perform a thorough neurologic exam including a mental status exam. If this exam is entirely normal and there is no sign of depressed or penetrating injury, the CT can be deferred in our current opinion. Continued observation and the ability to act on deterioration are mandatory.

This case is probably not one of parental abuse. Only one feature, the situation of a fall from the top bunk, suggests it. Child abuse ("child battering" or "nonaccidental trauma") may account for up to 30% of fractures, burns, and head injuries in young children. The physician's suspicions should be aroused by an injury that is inconsistent with the reported trauma; an inordinate delay in bringing the child to medical attention; prior injuries to the child or a sibling; the child's failure to thrive; and bizarre injuries (in this case for example, one must ask what a 2-year-old child was doing on a top bunk).

Parents of battered children usually have a history of beating for discipline, but they rarely use one medical facility regularly. There may be a family crisis, perhaps a very small one, and no source of help, and the parents take out their hostility on the child. Long-bone x-rays and skull films often reveal many new and old fractures. Bruises in different stages of healing, scald burns to the buttocks, and cigarette burns are also typical patterns of abuse. It is usually not a good idea for the emergency physician to accuse the family of child abuse. We urge early involvement of the pediatric staff physician and social workers.

The child may need hospitalization for protection even if this is not warranted by the severity of his injuries. Any suspicion of child abuse must always be reported to the appropriate agency as mandated by law.

The physician may either feel contempt for the injured child's family or despair of effecting any change in their treatment of the child, but neither attitude is warranted. Child-battering parents were usually battered or neglected children themselves, and only by supporting and encouraging them can agencies help them change their pattern of child-rearing. The physician's hostility may drive them "underground" and thus away from sources of help to which the pediatrics department might refer them.

REFERENCES
Textbook   Rosen. Pp. 377–393.

Review Article   Weeks, L. E. Handling of non-severe head injuries. *J.A.C.E.P.* 1979;8:257.

Additional   Feuerman, T., et al. Value of skull radiography, head computed
References   tomagraphic scanning, and admission for observation in cases of minor head injury. *Neurosurgery* 1988;22:449–453.

Freed, H. Post-traumatic skull films: Who needs them? *Ann. Emerg. Med.* 1986;15:233–235.

Chadwick, D.L. Child Abuse. In A.M. Rudolph (ed.), *Pediatrics* (18th ed.). East Norwalk, CT: Appleton and Lange, 1987. Pp. 760–769.

Case 66 Pregnant and Bleeding

A 17-year-old woman came to the emergency department complaining of vaginal spotting since four hours earlier that morning. She was four months pregnant and had already been seen twice in the obstetrics clinic. This was her first pregnancy, and she very much wanted the baby. Early in the pregnancy she had suffered with nausea and vomiting; otherwise, she was well. Her past history was uneventful except for an allergy to penicillin. This day she had lost about 2 teaspoonfuls of blood vaginally and was quite concerned.

The examining physician found the patient in bed, holding tightly to her young husband's hand. Her vital signs included blood pressure 120/72 supine and 110/50 seated, pulse 80 supine or seated, and temperature 36.2°C orally. Head, eyes, and throat were normal. Her chest was clear. Her abdomen showed slight tenderness throughout and a uterus halfway between pubis and umbilicus. A pelvic exam by speculum was done and disclosed a blue cervix with a closed os. There was no inordinate tenderness.

How often does bleeding occur in pregnancy?

Is it ever dangerous to do a pelvic exam in such a setting?

What is wrong with this young woman, and what should be done?

DISCUSSION   Bleeding is common in pregnancy, occurring in perhaps a third
of pregnancies, even those that go on to a healthy, full-term
delivery. The significance of the bleeding varies depending on
the stage of pregnancy.

We see a fair number of women with incomplete abortions in
the first trimester. Such patients will have significant bleeding,
usually more than their usual quantity for a menstrual period,
or will pass actual tissue other than blood. We examine such
patients, and, if the cervical os is open and there is active bleeding from the os, they are admitted for ultrasound and possible
dilatation and curettage. If the os is closed and the bleeding is
minimal, they can be followed as outpatients by their attending
obstetrician or the obstetrical clinic. We draw a baseline hematocrit and a serum human chorionic gonadotropin level at the
time of the visit and advise that the patient avoid sexual activity
and strenuous exertion until followup. Cultures are also obtained for chlamydia and gonorrhea. If adnexal tenderness or a
mass is palpated, a pelvic ultrasound is performed to verify that
the pregnancy is in the uterus. If no intrauterine pregnancy is
found on ultrasound, the patient is admitted to be worked up
for an ectopic pregnancy.

Once into the second trimester, abortions are much less frequent. This patient probably has less than a 10% chance of
completing an abortion. She is said to have a threatened abortion and will be reassured and sent home. She should be told to
return if she begins to pass copious amounts (more than
enough to use one sanitary pad per hour) of blood or tissue or
to have severe pain. She should avoid intercourse and douching
(no douching ever during pregnancy). She should be seen
again in any case at the obstetrics clinic within one month.

If bleeding occurs in the last half of the pregnancy, we advise
not doing a pelvic exam in the ED. A placenta previa or abrup-
tio may be present, and examination might increase the chance
of losing the fetus. Of course, copious bleeding may require us
to start several intravenous routes, give quantities of fluid, and
type and crossmatch and perhaps transfuse many units of
blood.

If the patient is hemorrhaging vigorously, her life takes precedence and a pelvic exam should be done. If possible this should
be done in the operating room in case emergency cesarean
section is necessary. Sometimes the products of conception are
found in the cervical os, and simple removal quiets down the
bleeding. When the bleeding is so severe as to force a pelvic
exam, it should, of course, begin with a careful speculum exam-

ination, which has less chance than a bimanual exam of disturbing a placenta previa. Ultrasound too is available and useful in diagnosing such pathology as placenta previa, and should be used when the bleeding is not life-threatening and there is time to review the situation more closely.

The thoroughness of the physician's examination, his or her explanation of the patient's symptoms, and reassurance that the pregnancy is a normal one are most important here. It is not enough for the physician to be assured that nothing is wrong; he or she must convey this feeling to the patient also.

REFERENCES

Textbook   Tintinalli. Pp. 396–398.

Review Article   Sinkinson, C. A., and Baker, D. T. The complaint of vaginal bleeding during pregnancy: A double dose of anxiety. *Emerg. Med. Rep.* 1989;10(1):1–8.

Additional   Gilling-Smith, G., et al. Management of early pregnancy bleed-
Reference   ing in the accident and emergency department. *Arch. Emerg. Med.* 1988;5:133–138.

Case 67 Trouble Breathing

A 52-year-old man came to the emergency department complaining of difficulty getting his breath. He had been troubled with shortness of breath for the previous two weeks, but it had become even worse today. He said that he had asthma.

The man had smoked two packs of cigarettes a day for many years and had a total smoking history of over sixty pack-years. He had quit smoking six months earlier on discharge from the state penitentiary where he had been a prisoner for nine years. He did not wish to discuss the cause of his incarceration. Shortness of breath had become noticeable about age 40 and was more and more frequently a problem during the past year. He had been told while in prison that he had asthma and had been treated with a combination drug containing ephedrine, theophylline, and a barbiturate. At times he had been on corticosteroids and used a bronchodilator inhaler.

During the past two years the patient had been bothered by a cough usually productive of a few ounces of yellow sputum daily. In fact, when pressed, he admitted to a "cigarette cough" most mornings of the past ten years. The cough was worse in the past few days, and the sputum was becoming darker, a sort of grayish green in color. During the past six months he had never been free of cough and could never walk more than three blocks without having to stop to get his breath. The preceding night he was up most of the night with coughing and difficulty getting his breath.

On examination the patient was observed to be having difficulty breathing. He appeared fatigued and could say no more than a few words at a time between breaths. His chest was hyperexpanded, and he took a long time with each breath. Vital signs included blood pressure 160/90, pulse 90, respiration 24, jugular venous pressure elevated in expiration but normal in inspiration, and temperature 37.0°C orally. His breath sounds were altered: One could not hear any normal alveolar breath sounds, but he did have high-pitched wheezes bilaterally. His heart was best heard in the epigastrium, and the heart tones were normal. His liver was low, with an upper edge percussible at almost the costal margin but with a total height in the mid-clavicular line of only 11 centimeters. There was no edema, and the rest of the examination showed no abnormalities.

Does this man have asthma?

What sort of problems lead to the appearance of such a patient at the ED?

What can be done for him?

DISCUSSION   Most middle-aged or older patients who arrive at the ED with the comment that their asthma is getting worse do not have asthma. A few of them have severe congestive heart failure, even pulmonary edema. These can often be diagnosed by the presence of edema, hepatomegaly, and above all an elevated venous pressure. These patients with pulmonary edema may have no rales but rather a chest full of musical wheezes, hence the term *cardiac asthma*. The history may include episodes of paroxysmal nocturnal dyspnea occurring two to four hours after going to bed, aiding diagnosis.

More often, as in this case, the older patient who labels himself as asthmatic has a chronic obstructive lung disease of the emphysema-bronchitis type. He may present with a history primarily of dyspnea for many years, may be oxygenated but wasted, and can be described as a "pink puffer." Such a patient usually can be kept out of the hospital until his ultimate decline and thus never accumulates a large inpatient chart. The patient suffering from relatively pure emphysema is less common than the bronchitic patient who describes years of cough before he developed significant dyspnea and often appears cyanotic. This "blue bloater" arrives frequently at the ED with the complications of infection (worsening bronchitis, pneumonia, or bronchiolitis), heart failure, mechanical disasters (pneumothorax, enlarging bleb restricting the vital capacity), or pulmonary emboli. Such a patient thus has many hospital admissions and typically has several volumes to his medical record.

This patient has characteristics both of emphysema and of bronchitis. He may also have some airway narrowing that will respond to bronchodilators and is therefore termed *reversible*. In the ED we treat him with low-flow oxygen, an intravenous loading dose infusion of 5 to 6 mg per kg of aminophylline, and inhaled bronchodilators such as metaproterenol or albuterol. We obtain baseline lab data including CBC, chest x-ray, ECG, and arterial blood gases. We look at the sputum for white blood cells and bacteria. It is seldom helpful to culture sputum unless the chest x-ray shows a pneumonia. Occasionally we can discharge such a patient on antibiotics (we prefer sulfamethoxazole/trimethoprim or ampicillin), but usually we are obliged to admit him for further evaluation and therapy.

One of the most vexing problems that faces the ED physician in treating the patient with chronic obstructive pulmonary disease is the decision to initiate mechanical ventilation. Such a decision depends on the physician's judgement and also the patient's wishes. Certain warning signs or signals should prompt the physician to think of mechanical ventilation with these patients. First and foremost is the patient's clinical presentation. If he is unable to speak more than one or two words without gasping, seems to have an altered mental status, or on lung exam is moving very little air, the chances that he will need mechanical ventilation are very good. In addition, if, despite appropriate therapy, the patient's respiratory acidosis is worsening because of increasing retained carbon dioxide, mechanical ventilation may be needed. Remember that it is difficult to judge the need for intubation based on the result of one arterial blood gas. Some patients with chronic obstructive pulmonary disease (COPD) are chronically hypoxemic with pO_2's between 40 and 50 and pCO_2's between 50 and 60 even during their compensated periods; however, these patients are generally not acidotic and will not show evidence of acute decompensation on initial examination. More important are serial results from blood gases, which give a very good indication as to whether the patient is improving or worsening.

We hesitate to intubate the COPD patient because it is often very difficult or impossible to wean him from the ventilator. Intubation of these patients should not be undertaken lightly. Nevertheless, mechanical ventilation may be needed only temporarily and can be lifesaving, thus provoking a very difficult clinical decision. If the patient is tiring and desires intubation, it should be performed.

REFERENCES

Textbook   Tintinalli. Pp. 284–288.

Review Article   Fanta, C. H., and Ingram, R. H. Chronic Obstructive Diseases of the Lung. In E. Rubenstein and D. D. Federman (eds.), *Scientific American Medicine.* 1989;14;III:1–22.

Additional   Nicotra, M. B., Reveria, M., and Awer, J. A. Antibiotic therapy
Reference   of acute exacerbations of chronic bronchitis. *Ann. Intern. Med.* 1982;97:18–21.

Case 68 Gunshot Wound

A 33-year-old man was brought to the emergency department by ambulance. He had been despondent and had attempted suicide by shooting himself with a .38-caliber revolver. The bullet entered two intercostal spaces below the left nipple and exited at the left posterior axillary line in the tenth intercostal space.

On arrival at the ED, the patient was conscious and breathing. He had a palpable systolic blood pressure of 60 mm Hg. His cardiac rate was 130 per minute. Three large intravenous infusions were begun with lactated Ringer's solution. A right internal jugular line and two antecubital fossa lines were placed with large-diameter short intracatheters. Within five minutes 500 ml of fluid had been given, and his blood pressure was palpable and audible at 100 mm Hg. A single chest tube was placed in the left midaxillary line in the fifth interspace. The pectoralis major muscle was grasped and the tube placed just posterior to it. The tube was connected to underwater drainage and then via a three-bottle system to continuous suction. Less than 100 ml of blood returned via the chest tube.

A Foley indwelling bladder catheter and a nasogastric tube were placed. A portable chest x-ray was taken. It showed a normal chest and a metal fragment probably below the diaphragm. The patient was told he needed an operation, and within thirty minutes of his arrival at the ED he was moved into the operating room. At that time the central venous pressure readings from his jugular vein catheter were about 14 centimeters. Eight units of blood were readied, he was intubated and anesthetized, and his abdomen was opened.

The laparotomy exposed about 1000 ml of free blood in the peritoneal cavity, a bisected spleen, and tears in the stomach and the jejunum. As the spleen was being removed, the patient's blood pressure became unobtainable despite a CVP of 18 centimeters. The chest was then opened, and a bulging pericardium was incised. A large amount of clot was easily evacuated, and a tangential crease wound of the apex of the heart was reinforced with sutures. The blood pressure rose on opening

the pericardium, and the rest of the operation proceeded uneventfully.

When and how should chest tubes be placed?

When should a traumatized patient have his chest opened in
the ED?

Is there any value to needle pericardiocentesis in a traumatic
hemopericardium?

DISCUSSION   Penetrating thoracic trauma can produce the following life-threatening injuries: tension pneumothorax, heart or great vessel injury with exsanguination, pericardial tamponade, and intra-abdominal hemorrhage. Initial treatment of the patient centers, of course, on the ABCs. Endotracheal intubation should be undertaken early if there are signs of airway compromise. At least two large-bore intravenous lines should be established even if the patient appears to be stable on initial assessment. If the patient is unstable on presentation, three or four peripheral intravenous lines and a large-bore central line should be placed, and blood for type and crossmatch and initial hematocrit should be sent immediately. Patients who present in shock can be transfused with O-negative or type-specific, uncrossmatched blood.

Tension pneumothorax is a deadly cause of hypotension in penetrating thoracic trauma. It causes displacement of the mediastinal structures followed by decreased cardiac output and cardiovascular collapse. Treatment is immediate decompression of the chest with a large-bore intravenous catheter placed in the second intercostal space at the midclavicular line. This should always be followed by insertion of a thoracostomy tube, as needle decompression is only a temporizing measure. Because this entity can be rapidly fatal, immediate action is necessary when it is clinically suspected. An x-ray study of the chest may cause a disastrous delay in patient care. Sucking (open) chest wounds should be temporarily sealed with a petrolatum gauze (such as Xeroform) taped on three sides to let air escape if under pressure but not be drawn into the chest cavity.

We feel rather free to place chest tubes. Any traumatized patient who is dyspneic, tachypneic, or in whom we clinically suspect a pneumothorax or hemothorax may get one or two chest tubes placed even before the five minutes it would take to obtain a portable x-ray of the chest. Physical findings of the chest may be nonrevealing and easily confused since listening to breath sounds and percussion can be suboptimal in a busy trauma room. A serious hemothorax may be missed by relying on auscultation. Chest tubes are fairly benign considering the tremendous potential danger of the patient's basic problems.

We prefer one tube in the fourth or fifth intercostal space between the anterior axillary and midaxillary lines. If the patient is awake, we try to anesthetize the skin and perichondrium with about 10 ml of 1% lidocaine, make a 1-inch long incision in the skin, separate deeper layers down to and including the parietal pleura with a large clamp or spreading movements of a pair of scissors, and then probe the wound with a gloved finger. If the finger tells you that you are in the chest cavity, a large chest tube is placed by grasping its tip in a large curved surgical clamp and advancing it over your probing finger. Tubes have been mistakenly placed below the diaphragm. This does no good and may damage the liver or spleen, so we try to avoid it. Occasionally a chest tube is placed on the wrong side (appearing correct until it is observed that the bullet's trajectory was bizarre and led to contralateral damage). If in doubt or if the patient is not improving, we do not hesitate to place a tube on the other side.

Penetrating injuries to the chest that damage the great vessels can be rapidly fatal. The majority of patients sustaining such injuries do not reach the ED alive. Stab wounds are usually less serious than gunshot wounds. The patient with heart or great vessel injury usually presents in hemorrhagic shock. Fluid resuscitation and rapid diagnosis of cardiac or great vessel injury are necessary for salvage. Findings that indicate the possibility of cardiac or great vessel injury include persistent hypotension and evidence of pericardial tamponade. Even when tamponade is found to be present, needle pericardiocentesis may be of very little value. It frequently returns nothing even when much blood has clotted in the pericardium and led to cardiac tamponade. Search for a paradoxical pulse is useless. This sign, defined in a spontaneously breathing patient with resting respiration, is grossly distorted in a patient who is in respiratory distress and totally obviated in one who is receiving positive pressure ventilation. The only useful signs are hypotension and a high or rising central venous pressure. It is possible to plug a myocardial rent with a finger or intraventricular Foley catheter balloon as a holding maneuver until the operating room's greater resources can be reached. In this most dramatic situation, one who hesitates is lost. Life-threatening hypotension following penetrating chest trauma may be due to cardiac tamponade, and after a brief but vigorous search for other sources of blood loss, the heart should be attacked directly. Sometimes this must be done in the ED. Emergency thoracotomy in the operating room is indicated for patients who continue to have hypotension despite aggressive fluid resuscitation, have an initial chest tube output of greater than 1000 ml of blood, have more than 250 ml of blood output in two consecutive hours, or have other signs of cardiac or great vessel injury. ED thoracotomy is indicated in patients who are victims of penetrating chest or abdominal trauma and died en route to or while in the ED.

In this case the initial approach failed to turn up an intra-thoracic cause for the patient's hypotension. The surgeon knew that the diaphragm can rise to the fourth intercostal space during expiration. The next obvious place to look was his abdomen, and it was quickly opened; however, the more serious disturbance was intrathoracic, and it was treated appropriately. If he had not responded promptly in the ED, a thoracotomy could have been done there. Nevertheless, the best place for these maneuvers is still a well-equipped and well-lighted operating room.

Prehospital care of these patients should be aimed toward rapid transport to the nearest trauma center. This "scoop and run" approach should include as much stabilization with peripheral intravenous lines, MAST trousers, and airway control as the paramedics are able to accomplish en route to the hospital. The caveat on the streets is that field care should not delay transport to the hospital.

REFERENCES

Textbook   Tintinalli. Pp. 850–863.

Review Article   Karrel, R., Shaffer, M. A., and Franszek, J. B. Emergency diagnosis, resuscitation and treatment of acute penetrating cardiac trauma. *Ann. Emerg. Med.* 1982;11:504–517.

Additional References   Hoffman, J. R. Emergency department thoracotomy. *Ann. Emerg. Med.* 1981;10:275–278.

Ordog, D. J. Emergency thoracotomy. *Am. J. Emerg. Med.* 1987;
5:312–316.

Fackner, M. L. Ballistic injury. *Ann. Emerg. Med.* 1986;15:1451–1455.

Case 69 Pleuritic Pain

A 65-year-old man came to the emergency department complaining of chest pain. He said the pain in his right side had begun about twenty-four hours earlier and had been getting worse since then. It was constantly present but excruciating when he coughed or moved suddenly. He was most comfortable sitting quietly or lying on his right side. Although he denied smoking or drinking, he did admit to a cough the preceding few days that produced a small amount of yellow sputum. Prior to this illness he had been quite well and active and denied any chronic cough, prior chest pains, or shortness of breath.

On physical examination the patient appeared well. His vital signs included blood pressure 150/80, pulse 100, respiration 20, temperature 38.3°C orally, and a normal jugular venous pressure. His head, eyes, ears, nose, and throat were unremarkable. His neck was carefully palpated, revealing no adenopathy or other pathology. His chest was slightly tender laterally on the right side, and there were a few crackling rales audible there. His cardiovascular examination was normal; he had no edema; and the rest of the exam showed nothing remarkable. A chest x-ray showed a right lower lobe infiltrate involving almost the entire lobe.

What is the diagnosis in this case?

What further studies should be done?

What should be done for this man?

DISCUSSION This man seems to have a pneumonia, and most pneumonias are pneumococcal. Alcoholics, postinfluenza patients, diabetics, and the like all usually have the pneumococcus as causative organism when they develop a bacterial pneumonia.

After pneumococcus, the next most likely cause of pneumonia acquired in the community is mycoplasma. Mycoplasma most commonly occurs in the 10- to 30-year age group. The illness it causes is usually more gradual than pneumococcus in onset. Symptoms include fatigue, headache, myalgias, and a nonproductive hacking cough. Pleuritic chest pain and fever greater than 102°F (38.9°C) are unusual. In contrast, pneumococcal pneumonia often produces pleuritic chest pain, a cough productive of purulent sputum, chills, and temperature elevations exceeding 102°F. If the patient is immunocompromised by the human immunodeficiency virus, the most common pneumonia is caused by *Pneumocystis carinii*. Previously a rare disorder, *Pneumocystis carinii* pneumonia (PCP) has grown to an epidemic along with the acquired immunodeficiency syndrome.

The two most important procedures in confirming the presence of pneumonia are the chest x-ray and sputum gram stain. We recommend obtaining one or two blood cultures prior to initiating therapy since blood cultures are frequently positive in pneumococcal pneumonia and may confirm the diagnosis when sputum cultures are negative. The white blood cell count, erythrocyte sedimentation rate, and the c-reactive protein are usually elevated in patients with bacteremia, but these tests provide only minimal additional information. When a good sputum smear is examined, it will often show a preponderance of one organism. If this is indeed a gram-positive diplococcus, therapy should be begun with penicillin. Care must be taken to obtain sputum, not saliva. This patient (if not allergic to penicillin) could be given 2.4 million units of procaine penicillin G intramuscularly followed by 500 mg of penicillin V orally qid.

Because our bed capacity is limited, we often are not able to admit patients with pneumonia to the hospital. Many do well at home. These outpatient regimens need careful monitoring. The patient must return in two or three days, sooner if he is worse. The patients who have lowered host resistance or appear very ill should be admitted to the hospital. Any alcoholic or diabetic with pneumonia needs hospitalization as do pregnant or dehydrated patients and those for whom adequate followup cannot be assured. Most patients over age 50 should be admitted. The presence of a high fever, tachypnea, severe chest pain, or hypoxia argues for admission.

The differential diagnosis of this patient included all of the other conditions that commonly can present with the sudden onset of severe respiratory chest pain: spontaneous pneumothorax, pleurodynia (a "viral pleurisy"), pulmonary embolism, pericarditis, and bronchitis with chest wall injury from coughing.

This patient was treated at home, and he improved rapidly. When seen again in three days, he felt much better and was afebrile. In two weeks his chest x-ray was normal and he had returned to normal.

REFERENCES

Textbook   Rosen. Pp. 1103–1117.

Review Article   Hopkins, C. G. Community Acquired Pneumonia. In A. P. Fishman (ed.), *Pulmonary Diseases and Disorders*, 2nd edition. New York, McGraw-Hill, 1988. Pp. 1535–1541.

Additional   The choice of antimicrobial drugs. *Med. Lett.* 1988;30:33–40.
References
                      MacFarlane, J. T. Treatment of lower respiratory infections. *Lancet* 1987;2(8573):1446–1449.

Case 70 Looked "Too Drunk" to the Police

A 38-year-old man was brought to the emergency department by city police. He had been arrested for being drunk in a public place and taken to the city jail. After seven hours in jail he had appeared "too drunk" to his jailers and was brought to the ED. Because no ED beds were available, the man was placed in the locked ED jail cell. A physician saw him within one hour of his arrival in the ED but quickly turned away. The patient was disheveled, malodorous, uncooperative, unshaven, ataxic, and appeared quite drunk. No careful neurologic or mental status exam was done, and he was left in the cell to sober up. When next seen three hours later, he was stuporous and had one large pupil. He was quickly taken from the cell, undressed, examined, and rushed to the operating room, where an epidural hematoma was evacuated. Despite these vigorous efforts the patient died on the operating table.

How can you tell that a patient is drunk?

How can you tell that he is *just* drunk?

Is it surprising that this man had no obvious signs of trauma and yet had an acute epidural hematoma?

Does an acute subdural hematoma also present this way?

DISCUSSION   Alcohol intoxication is a common pathologic state in most EDs. The features that should be looked for include slurred speech, a tendency to drift off to sleep, inappropriate behavior, and mild ataxia. A blood alcohol is helpful. A level of 100 mg per 100 ml is used in most states to define a patient as too drunk to drive; one is usually definitely ataxic at 200 mg per 100 ml, and stupor appears at about 300 mg per 100 ml in the occasional drinker. A chronic alcoholic (the "chronic" is redundant) may not become sleepy until a higher level—400 or 500 mg per 100 ml—due to central nervous system (CNS) tolerance to the alcohol. In this patient, who had been off alcohol for at least eight hours when first seen in the ED, a blood alcohol probably would have been under 100 mg per 100 ml. Such a low level would have alerted the physician to the presence of another problem.

The big problem is ruling out the existence of other pathology accompanying alcohol intoxication as cause of the ataxia or stupor. This patient was still "drunk" after seven hours of sobering up time, and the physician should have made a more careful search for other pathology. A patient with a blood alcohol of 400 mg per dl may also have a subdural hematoma, an epidural hematoma, cerebellar degeneration, or any other pathology. The examination should include vital signs (a wide pulse pressure or bradycardia may be the tip-off to rising intracranial pressure), gait, mentation, and a careful search for head trauma. It is very difficult to evaluate CNS disorders in a drunk patient. A careful search for any lateralizing sign is essential, as is a cervical spine x-ray series if trauma is being seriously considered. If any doubt remains about the possibility of an acute intracranial bleed, a CT scan should be done.

It is not surprising that there was no gross evidence of head trauma. Epidural hematomas often result from a relatively small trauma that hits at precisely the right spot to tear the middle meningeal artery. A baseball or hockey puck can do this. The patient with an acute subdural hematoma is more often the victim of more massive trauma: He was hit by a car or a truck rather than a baseball. As a result, he has multiple injuries, and since focal neurologic signs may be scant, we sometimes spend valuable time elsewhere before evaluating the cause of his confusion or unconsciousness. A chronic subdural hematoma often presents weeks after the trauma, and the patient may no longer give a history of any trauma. This disorder is replacing syphilis as "the great imitator" and should be thought of in any confused or sleepy patient. This is especially true if he is aged or an alcoholic, frequent settings for a chronic subdural hematoma.

REFERENCES

Textbook   Tintinalli. Pp. 829–845.

Review Article Galbraith, S. Misdiagnosis and delayed diagnosis in traumatic intracranial hematoma. *Br. Med. J.* 1976;1:1438–1439.

Additional   Macewen, W. The diagnosis of alcoholic coma. *Glasgow Med.*
References   *J.* 1879;1(January):1–15.

Jennett, B., et al. Severe head injuries in three countries. *J. Neurol. Neurosurg. Psychiatry* 1977;40:291–298.

Case 71 Aspirin plus Iron

A 20-year-old woman came to the emergency department after she had taken twenty to thirty Anacin tablets and an unknown quantity of iron capsules. She had already vomited spontaneously and appeared somewhat anxious. Since her physical exam revealed nothing unusual, she was observed for two hours and sent home. She returned the next day confused and complaining of persistent vomiting and hematemesis. Her stomach was distended and contained over 1500 ml of bloody material. In addition, she was hypotensive—her reclining blood pressure was 90/60 and dropped 20 mm when she sat up. Her BUN was 48. The patient was admitted to the hospital, and she improved with subsequent care, which included psychiatric treatment.

What was the problem here?

What other drugs are more dangerous than would be initially apparent when taken in overdoses?

Case 71 was adapted from Platt, F. W., Ironclad problem. *Emerg. Med.* 1972;4:165.

DISCUSSION   The severity of aspirin and iron intoxication in adults is often underestimated. The danger cannot be measured in terms of coma, as it can after the ingestion of many other, more often ingested substances. Iron can produce a severe hemorrhagic gastritis that can lead to death and may be treated with desferoxamine, a highly specific chelator of ferric iron. Aspirin produces a series of severe metabolic disturbances that may culminate in a metabolic acidosis or a respiratory alkalosis. Thorough initial evaluation should include arterial blood gas studies and evaluation of the patient's metabolic status before discharge.

The other drug overdoses we most often see underappreciated in our ED are the antidepressants, which may well present with a conscious patient and yet lead to fatal arrhythmias an hour after ingestion.

Some potentially severe overdoses will show apparent early recovery, as with iron, or an initial lack of worrisome symptoms, as with acetaminophen. Acetaminophen overdose can produce a fatal hepatotoxicity which will manifest itself days after the asymptomatic overdose itself.

Poison control centers provide first-aid telephone advice to the general public and more detailed information to inquiring medical personnel. Ideally the phones are staffed by pharmacists, doctors of pharmacology, and physicians, with a toxicologist available. As the initial reference many EDs use the Poisindex system. It is an expensive but reliable microfiche system published by the Rocky Mountain Poison Center and updated quarterly.

REFERENCES
Textbook   Rosen. Pp. 2141–2149, 2193–2202.

Review Articles Snodgrass, W. Salicylate toxicity. *Pediatr. Clin. North Am.* 1986; 33:381–392.

Banner, R. W., and Tong, T. G. Iron poisoning. *Pediatr. Clin. North Am.* 1986;33:393–409.

Additional   Platt, F. W. Ironclad problems. *Emerg. Med.* 1972;4:165.
References
Schauben, J. L., et al. Iron poisoning: Report of three cases and a review of therapeutic intervention. *J. Emerg. Med.* 1990;8:309–319.

Case 72 No Pulse

A 55-year-old man was brought to the emergency department by ambulance. He was complaining of abdominal pain. As he was wheeled into the ED, the ambulance attendant mentioned that he had been unable to feel a pulse. The patient was immediately surrounded by a group of physicians and nurses, who noted that he was apparently conscious and communicating but indeed had no obtainable blood pressure and no obtainable peripheral pulses. His carotid pulse was palpable and his heart rate 110. There were several long scars on his chest, abdomen, and legs. An ECG showed a broad QRS with a duration of 0.16 second and a regular rate of 110. No P waves were evident. A central venous pressure line was placed, and it read 28 centimeters. The physician's initial impression was probably tempered by his just having been involved in a case of dissecting aortic aneurysm in which the diagnosis had initially been missed. It was difficult to avoid the same diagnosis in this case.

A call to the patient's regular physician revealed that this man had undergone extensive vascular surgery including myocardial revascularization in the past two years. He had shown no palpable pulses for many months. The ECG was then reviewed, and the diagnosis of hyperkalemia was made. Therapy was begun with glucose, insulin, and sodium bicarbonate. Serum potassium level was 6.8 mEq per liter.

What is the usual first therapy given to a pulseless patient?

What are the ECG findings of hyperkalemia?

What are the usual causes of hyperkalemia?

DISCUSSION   A pulseless patient usually is assumed to be in ventricular fibrillation and greeted immediately with a very quick evaluation
of the ABCs (Airway, Breathing, and Circulation) followed by
cardiopulmonary resuscitation and a direct current shock of
200 watt seconds. This is done even before a diagnostic ECG.
Occasionally such a patient will be in severe shock, and there is
indeed a possibility that a defibrillation will result in fibrillation
rather than cure it. Even more rarely, as in this case, the pulseless patient will show evidence of adequate cardiac output
(such as retaining consciousness), leading us to defer electro-
shock.

Extensive peripheral vascular disease in combination with hypotension and vasoconstriction may lead to poorly palpable
pulses. Severe shock of any cause or dissection of the aorta
with or without aneurysm formation may also lead to poor
peripheral perfusion without palpable pulses. Of course if the
patient is not awake, management proceeds according to Advanced Cardiac Life Support (ACLS) protocols depending on
the presenting rhythm, i.e., ventricular fibrillation, asystole, and
so forth.

Any adult patient with lower back pain, abdominal pain radiating to the back or groin, a pulsatile mass (particularly in the
epigastrium), or shock must be suspected of having an abdominal aortic aneurysm. Chest pain of a tearing nature radiating to
the back is typical of a dissecting thoracic aortic aneurysm.
Signs include unequal pulses, neurologic dysfunction, hemothorax, and ECG changes. In this same patient population, severe atherosclerosis may also affect the mesenteric vessels producing intestinal ischemia or infarction. Intestinal angina, a
syndrome of abdominal pain following meals, is a warning sign
of an impending mesenteric artery obstruction. The pain of a
bowel infarction is usually out of proportion to the amount of
tenderness found. The patient will complain of great pain but
have an "unimpressive" abdominal exam, thus often deceiving
the physician and delaying the diagnosis until it is too late.

Hyperkalemia (which was the diagnosis in this patient) usually first leads to peaked T waves and lengthening of the PR
interval. More severe hyperkalemia may cause loss of P wave,
widening of the QRS, and eventually a sine wave pattern easily
mistaken for ventricular flutter or tachycardia. Hyperkalemia
has two main causes: acidosis or uremia. This patient did indeed have renal failure, which led to both acidosis and uremia.
Potassium therapy can of course worsen either of these.

REFERENCES

Textbook   Rosen. Pp. 1983–1987.

Review Article   Dittrich, K. L., and Walls, R. M. Hyperkalemia: ECG manifesta-
                        tions and clinical considerations. *J. Emerg. Med.* 1986;4:449–
                        455.

Additional   Lee, K. S., Powell, B. L., and Adams, P. L. Focal neurologic
Reference   signs associated with hyperkalemia. *South. Med. J.* 1984;77:
                        792–793.

Case 73 Three Days of Cough/Cyanotic

A 34-year-old man collapsed just outside the emergency department. His friend told of a three-day course of progressive cough and fatigue. The patient had been well previously and was not on any medication. He was hypotensive, grossly cyanotic, and had a sinus tachycardia of 140 beats per minute. His breathing was shallow at about 30 respirations per minute, and he had bilateral rales and rhonchi. His venous pressure was not elevated, and he had no edema. Oxygen therapy was begun but held to 4 liters per minute because the attending physician was concerned about the possible danger of high-flow oxygen. An arterial blood sample showed a pO_2 of 40 mm Hg that produced a saturation of less than 70%. A chest film showed multiple large infiltrates thought to be pneumonia. Increasing the nasal oxygen flow to 12 liters per minute raised the oxygen saturation to 80%.

How much oxygen does one give a patient?

When should intubation be performed?

Case 73 was adapted from Platt, F. W., Enough is not too much. *Emerg. Med.* 1972;4:46.

DISCUSSION   This patient was in an advanced stage of acute respiratory failure. The early stages are characterized by dyspnea and an increase in the pulse, respiratory rate, and blood pressure. As the
respirations become more labored, the partial pressure of carbon dioxide increases and the patient begins to tire. Soon the
ventilations become more shallow and the patient's mental status changes. Untreated respiratory failure will then progress to
unconsciousness and death if not immediately treated.

Assisting the patient's ventilations with a bag-valve-mask will
do more than applying nasal oxygen. At 4 liters per minute, a
nasal cannula will increase the inspired oxygen fraction by
about 12 to 16%. Increasing the oxygen level to 12 liters per
minute will only increase the oxygen by about 20%. A nonrebreather mask with 10 to 15 liters per minute oxygen flow
would be more appropriate in this patient. This level of flow
provides almost 100% oxygen concentration.

The critical factor in oxygen therapy is to give enough oxygen. Even though some patients with chronic obstructive lung
disease cannot tolerate uncontrolled high-flow oxygen, they
need highflow oxygen, perhaps with the use of a ventilator.

In adults, the only contraindication to high-flow oxygen therapy is in the subset of COPD patients who are CO_2 retainers.
We give oxygen when it is desperately needed. If we do not
know whether or not the patient is a CO_2 retainer, we watch the
patient very closely for signs of respiratory depression. In some
cases, a Venturi mask can fine-tune the amount of oxygen flow
and help give the needed therapy while avoiding intubation.
Oxygen therapy should never be withheld or kept to a low flow
when the patient is dangerously hypoxic simply because the
physician is afraid of giving too much oxygen.

We see similar reluctance to give enough of an appropriate
therapy in many situations. Patients in shock are given inadequate volumes of intravenous fluids, agitated withdrawing alcoholics are given too little sedation, and patients in pain are
given too little analgesia. Too much of a good thing may be
bad, but too little can be too.

Intubation should be considered in any patient who is in
imminent respiratory failure. Signs of this include evidence of
overwhelming fatigue, falling blood pressure and pulse, and
alterations in mental status. If these are present, the patient
should be intubated. When these patients stop responding to
spoken voice, our experience is that you have about 1 minute
more before cardiac arrest occurs. Adequate ventilation is the
only preventative measure. Intubation can be done through the

nose if the patient has a gag reflex and an adequate tidal volume, otherwise it should be done orally.

REFERENCES

Textbook   Tintinalli. Pp. 249–252.

Review Article   Rosen, R. L. Acute respiratory failure and chronic lung disease. *Med. Clin. North Am.* 1986;70:895–907.

Additional   Carden, D. L., and Smith, J. K. Pneumonias. *Emerg. Med. Clin.*
Reference   *North Am.* 1989;7:255–278.

Case 74 Seizure

A 40-year-old man was brought to the emergency department because he had been found lying on the street unconscious. Shortly after his arrival, he had a five-minute major motor seizure. He was lying on a cart in the hall while a room was being readied for him when he had the fit. He was observed by several patients as well as their relatives and friends, two persons from housekeeping, two clerks, a policeman, and a nurse. The consternation was considerable among this group. The nurse found a physician and urged him to give the patient an injection of 10 mg of diazepam (Valium), which she handed him. The injection went in as the seizure was ending, to the great relief of the many observers. The patient was then given a brief physical examination that disclosed only stupor with no focal neurologic findings. He then was given 120 mg of phenobarbital intramuscularly. One hour later he was arousable enough to tell his story. He told of a seizure disorder of many years' standing but said he had recently stopped taking his usual phenytoin (Dilantin) to see what would happen.

When a patient has a seizure in the ED, how many has he probably had that day?

How do seizure patients present in the ED, and how should they be treated?

DISCUSSION   Usually a seizure patient who has a fit in the ED is having the second one for that day—the first one brought him to the ED. Thus therapy is usually but not always appropriate. Adult seizure patients arriving at the ED can often be classified in four groups: (1) known seizure disorder, (2) alcoholic—withdrawal or "rum fits," (3) status, by definition: repeated seizures without awakening in the interim, and (4) first seizure. In general, a blood sugar sample should always be obtained, as close to ictus as possible. In a person on medication, it is helpful to know his anticonvulsant drug levels.

1. *Known seizure disorder.* A person with a known seizure disorder may have a breakthrough in his control; this may be spontaneous, associated with drug juggling, or associated with alcohol intake, phenothiazines, or sleep deprivation. The therapeutic Dilantin level is 10 to 20 µg per ml (20 to 30 µg is associated with nystagmus; 30 to 40 µg with dysarthria and ataxia, i.e., "drunk-like state"; above 40 µg with drowsiness). A patient who ran out of medications a few days ago should be given a loading dose of his proper medications, either orally or intravenously.

2. *Alcoholic.* Withdrawal seizure may be associated with early alcohol withdrawal signs and symptoms such as tremulousness, anxiety, fever, sweating, tachycardia, focal hallucinations, etc. This may occur while the patient is still drinking but tapering off. The term *rum fit* actually refers to withdrawal seizures and so is a misnomer. Alcohol withdrawal seizures tend to cluster over several hours. Other than protecting the airway and keeping the patient from hurting himself on the stretcher, we do not specifically treat withdrawal seizures. A careful neurologic exam looking for signs of head trauma and lateralizing signs is essential to avoid the pitfall of labeling an intoxicated patient with an epidural hematoma as simple alcohol withdrawal.

3. *Status.* This is a life-threatening disorder. Someone in a seizure can be first treated with intravenous diazepam (Valium) in 5- to 10-mg increments, but diazepam's two disadvantages are respiratory depression and recurrence of seizures within thirty minutes. Lorazepam (Ativan) in 2- to 4-mg increments up to 8 mg is as effective as diazepam in initial seizure treatment, lasts longer, and may cause less respiratory depression in young adults; but be prepared to intubate if respiratory depression occurs. The benzodiazepine is followed by thiamine and glucose (if not already given). The patient

whose seizure continues must be loaded with phenytoin (Dilantin). We give 13 to 18 mg per kg intravenously at a maximum rate of 50 mg per minute, preferably 40 mg per minute, in normal saline, using an infusion pump and micro filter. The heart rhythm should be monitored during such an infusion. If the patient is awake and can wait several hours for a therapeutic blood level, it is safer and often more efficient to give the loading amount in one or two oral doses, but this is not an option in a patient who is still in status. One can always stop status with general anesthesia, usually barbiturates. We try phenobarbital 120 mg intravenously before calling anesthesiology.

4. *First seizure in an adult.* This is usually a good reason for admission and a full neurologic workup to determine cause (toxic, metabolic, tumor, cardiovascular, subarachnoid hemorrhage, infection, etc.). A history is needed from observer and patient regarding first, warnings (aura)—visual hallucinations, olfactory hallucinations (funny or unpleasant smells), feeling of familiarity or strangeness, sensations or jerking in limbs; and second, the seizure itself—lip-smacking, verbalization, head and eyes turning, focal limb-jerking, tongue-biting, incontinence, generalized seizure. A postictal exam should be done. The sooner it is done the more likely it will be to disclose a deficit. Look for focal limb weakness, reflex asymmetry, unilateral Babinski's sign, dysphasic speech; in other words, any focal signs. The ED workup should include analysis of blood sugar, electrolytes, BUN, calcium, magnesium, ECG, and may also include toxicologic studies for agents such as cocaine, propoxyphene, and tricyclic antidepressants. A CT scan of the head is indicated for any patient with a first seizure, if there is any lateralizing neurologic sign, or if the patient is having seizures of unknown etiology or out of proportion to their prior pattern.

Pseudoseizures are a fairly common phenomena and sometimes are seen in known seizure patients. In a typical pseudoseizure, the tonic-colonic movement is asymmetric and there is no postictal somnolence. One can suspect a pseudoseizure if the patient blinks during the seizure when the eyelid is lightly touched or if the patient protects himself from threats. Metabolic acidosis and elevation of creatine phosphokinase (CPK) enzymes, found after true seizures, are absent in pseudoseizures.

Finally, it should be said that the Valium given to this patient was probably unnecessary and unhelpful. His seizure was due to end shortly, he was not in status epilepticus, and the drug treated his onlookers' anxiety more than the patient's seizure disorder.

REFERENCES

Textbook Rosen. Pp. 1751–1767.

Review Article Delgado-Escueta, A. V., et al. Current concepts in neurology: Management and status of epilepticus. *N. Engl. J. Med.* 1982; 306:1337–1340.

Additional References Jadoga, A. A., and Riggio, S. Nonconvulsive status epilepticus in adults. *Am. Emerg. J. Med.* 1988;6:250–254.

Hunter, R. A. Status epilepticus: History, incidence and problems. *Epilepsia* 1959–1960;1:162–188.

Turnbull, T. L., et al. Utility of laboratory studies in the emergency department patient with a new-onset seizure. *Ann. Emerg. Med.* 1990;19:373–377.

Case 75 Skull X-Rays

A 3-year-old boy was brought to the emergency department by his parents. He had fallen off a slide about an hour earlier and hit his head. He initially cried vigorously and then calmed down. The parents were very worried. They mentioned that he was their first and only child.

On examination, the child moved all extremities well, cried lustily when stimulated, and had no focal neurologic abnormalities. His fundi were hard to examine, since he kept moving his eyes, but they seemed normal. There was a small tender swelling high on his forehead, but no blood was seen behind the ears or tympanic membranes.

Skull films were taken and read as normal. The physician seemed saddened by these findings and told the parents they were normal with a very negative affect. The parents became more worried but agreed to observe the child closely that night.

How should "negative findings" such as a normal skull x-ray be presented to patients and families?

In general, when do you take skull x-rays?

DISCUSSION   Normal findings are good news and should be announced as
such. A patient should feel that his doctor is working for his
health, not for his diseases. This physician could better have
approached the parents with a statement such as "I have good
news for you. The x-rays are normal. Your boy does not have a
skull fracture. I'm sure you are as happy as I am to know that."

For years there has been some controversy about when to
order skull x-rays, and the Food and Drug Administration con-
vened a national consensus panel recently. According to the
panel, all head-injured patients can be sorted into one of three
groups: low, medium, and high risk. High-risk patients are those
with an acute neurosurgical emergency. They have focal neurologic signs, a decreasing or depressed level of consciousness, or
known skull penetration or depression. These patients need a
stat head CT scan or a stat neurosurgical consultation, or both.
The delay to get skull x-rays for one of these patients can be
fatal. The low-risk group patients have a normal mental status,
a normal neurologic exam, and no other signs or symptoms of
major injury. They may also have a scalp laceration or a small
hematoma, but these are not necessarily signs of major injury.
The low-risk group patients do not need skull x-rays. They need
careful observation and discharge with a head injury instruction
sheet both given and explained to a responsible observer. Patients
in the moderate-risk category are harder to evaluate. They have
one or more of the following: history of loss of consciousness,
vomiting, amnesia, unclear or unreliable history of injury, age
less than 2 years, alcohol intoxication, signs of basilar skull
fracture, possible skull penetration (e.g., assault with a screw-
driver), or possible depressed fracture (high-impact injury, e.g.,
baseball bat). The role of skull x-rays and head CT in this group
is unclear; clinical judgement is called for. When in doubt we
often go ahead and obtain skull x-rays or a head CT study.

REFERENCES
Textbook   Rosen. Pp. 377–393, 1753–1754.

Review Article   Masters, S. J., et al. Skull x-ray examination after head trauma.
N. Engl. J. Med. 1987;316:84–91.

Additional   Dacey, R. G., et al. Neurosurgical complications after appar-
References   ently minor head injury: Assessment of risk in a series of 610
patients. *J. Neurosurg.* 1986;65:203–210.

Freed, H. A. Post traumatic skull films: Who needs them? *Ann.
Emerg. Med.* 1986;15:233–235.

Case 76 Flank Pain

A 27-year-old man was brought to the emergency department by a good friend of his who was a third-year medical student. The patient had been well until two hours earlier, when he was suddenly seized by severe pain in his left flank. He said that the pain was the worst he had ever experienced, that it came and went, and that he felt weak and nauseated when the pain was present. On his arrival at the ED, the pain had been absent for over half an hour, and he felt a bit embarrassed at being there. His friend had already done a urinalysis and reported seeing many white blood cells and bacteria in the urine. The patient was afebrile, and his physical examination revealed nothing noteworthy. His friend thought that the diagnosis was pyelonephritis and that antibiotics were indicated; however, review of the urinalysis by a staff physician showed red blood cells instead of white blood cells.

What is the diagnosis in this case?

Why the confusion in doing the urinalysis?

What should be done for this patient?

DISCUSSION   This patient probably had ureteral colic. The story of sudden, varying, severe flank pain associated with hematuria suggests the presence of a stone in the ureter. Otherwise well persons may have episodes of ureteral colic, which is usually severe pain. The pain may be flank, groin, scrotal, or a combination of these. A woman may complain of vulva or vaginal pain. There is usually vesicle irritability with dysuria and frequency of urination when the stone is entering the bladder. This patient probably has passed the stone into his bladder at this time. Occasionally a kidney or a ureteral stone will present with abdominal or back pain, and the diagnosis may be hard to make in the 10 to 15% of cases in which red blood cells are not present in the urine.

Mistaking red blood cells for white is not a difficult error for a neophyte examining an unstained urine sediment. The identification of bacteria is almost impossible in an unstained sediment. Dust, debris, and amorphous crystals commonly oscillate in brownian movement and simulate bacteria. Only a gram stain, or better still a urine culture, will identify bacteriuria. Of course, obstructive urinary disease and infective urinary disease are closely associated. Significant bacteriuria may be present, and a urine culture would be appropriate.

If the patient is in severe pain, we start an intravenous line, give several hundred ml of fluids and intravenous morphine for pain. We obtain a BUN or creatinine, and if it is normal we often get an intravenous pyelogram (IVP). If he has fever or chills, extravasation of dye, a stone over 6 mm in diameter in the renal pelvis, or a nonfunctioning (totally obstructed) kidney, we usually admit him to the hospital. If pain control is adequate and the stone looks small enough to pass, the patient can be discharged. If he is sent home, we give him a strainer and tell him to strain his urine as we have been doing in the ED. Followup is usually with the primary doctor or a urologist within a week.

It is often helpful to give the patient the discharge instructions in the presence of the person who brought him in. Patients frequently forget much of what is told to them in the course of treatment. We always give patients a discharge instruction sheet written in plain English (not "medicalese") that explains the medications to be taken, possible side effects, and a referral for followup care. We also list the danger signs that would signal worsening of their condition and require them to come to the ED: in this case, any fever, chills, or increasing pain not relieved by oral analgesics.

This patient had an IVP that was normal except for slight dilation of the collecting system on the left. His friend became very upset when he heard that no antibiotics were to be given. When they left, the patient was reassured and his friend very anxious.

REFERENCES
Textbook   Rosen. Pp. 1563–1572.

Review Article   Roth, R. A., and Finlayson, B. *Stones: Clinical Management of Urolithiasis.* Baltimore, Williams & Wilkins, 1983. Pp. 441–445.

Additional   Zangerle, K. F., et al. Usefulness of abdominal flat plate radio-
Reference   graphs in patients with suspected uretheral calculi. *Ann. Emerg. Med.* 1985;14:316–319.

Case 77 Tricyclic Antidepressant Overdose

On Tuesday, a 23-year-old woman was brought in by a local rescue squad because of an alleged tricyclic antidepressant (TCA) overdose. The patient had been treated with imipramine one year before. The rescue squad said that on their last shift, Monday, they were called to the same woman because of a possible overdose, but she was acting normally and had no signs of any problem. She told them that she had taken her normal dose of medication, did not feel depressed, and wanted no further treatment. In fact, she felt so good that she now could easily see how to "solve all of her problems." Her parents, who were on the scene, told the paramedic that she looked and acted better than she had in years, and they supported their daughter in refusing treatment. At the Monday call, the paramedics allowed her to sign a form stating she was requesting to be discharged against medical advice (AMA). The next morning her parents found her very drowsy in bed. Her medications were all missing. The rescue squad initiated an intravenous line and gave her 30 ml of ipecac. She did not vomit en route to the hospital.

On admission to the emergency department she could be easily aroused but spoke with slurred speech. Her blood pressure was 100/60, pulse 124, and respirations 14. Her pupils were large and reactive, lungs were clear, heart sounds normal, and abdomen benign. Her deep tendon reflexes were depressed. She stated that she took all her pills about an hour previously and wanted to die.

The patient was initially uncooperative with therapy. Immediate gastric lavage was begun using a 36 French orogastric tube. Lavage continued for one-half hour until the fluid return was clear. Fifty grams of activated charcoal was then placed down the tube.

At this point, her blood pressure dropped to 80/60 and frequent premature ventricular contractions (PVCs) were seen on the monitor. A twelve-lead ECG showed a widened QRS of 0.14 seconds. She was given 100 mEq of $NaHCO_3$ and a liter of 0.5 normal saline over thirty minutes. This corrected the hypotension and the PVCs and her QRS complex duration dropped to 0.12 seconds.

On the way to the intensive care unit, she became agitated. She tried to jump off the stretcher and required physical restraints. Physostigmine 1 mg was given very slowly, and within a minute she began to calm but then had a sudden grand mal seizure and became asystolic. Full resuscitative efforts were unable to reverse this, and she was pronounced dead one hour after her cardiac arrest.

Should a patient be tied down and treated despite her refusal to give consent for such therapy?

What is the best initial treatment to empty the stomach in cases of massive overdose?

What went wrong here?

DISCUSSION   Reasonable therapeutic restraint is always proper in emergency medicine. This includes the prehospital care given to any patient. The EMTs on the scene cannot simply allow a patient to refuse medical treatment (sign out AMA). If a patient with any but the most minor illness or injury wishes to sign AMA, the EMTs should contact a medical control authority for assistance.

An AMA form is a potentially dangerous thing in an ED. It often allows poor therapy to be excused. A patient who refuses care for minor problems should have her refusal noted on her chart with a clear statement of the patient's mental status and the explanation that was given to her. If it is possibly a true emergency, however, she should be restrained and treated. Most patients will become cooperative when they realize that we will not take no for an answer.

This patient's refusal to accept treatment the first time she was seen by the paramedics suggests that she had formulated a plan to kill herself. Any depressed patient who suddenly states she is fine and has no further problems should be considered a high suicide risk.

A major evolving issue in the treatment of the overdose patient is how to empty the stomach. Syrup of ipecac is commonly used to induce emesis but can be dangerous. It should not be used in ingestions of severe caustics (acid or alkali), low-viscosity hydrocarbons (like gasoline), or in any patient who may develop a significantly depressed mental status. Finally, it must not be used when *rapid* gastric emptying is essential, such as in TCA overdose.

A large-bore Ewald-type stomach tube can be used for gastric lavage, although if the patient has an inadequate gag reflex or is lethargic, the airway needs to be protected first (i.e., intubate the patient before placing the Ewald tube). At least 2000 ml of water should be used in the lavage attempt. We fill and empty the stomach repeatedly with 400-ml amounts of saline or tap water. A small-bore nasogastric tube is of very little value in lavage as it will not easily return pill fragments.

Possibly even more valuable than lavage is the administration of a slurry of charcoal. If both ipecac and charcoal are used, the charcoal must be held until vomiting has occurred. Charcoal is often mixed with a cathartic to further decrease absorption of the ingested drug.

TCA overdoses are common. These drugs have strong anticholinergic properties, quinidine-like membrane stabilizing effects on cardiac cells, and they block the reuptake of norepinephrine. Clinically, the patient with TCA overdose may present with altered mental status, seizures, coma, hypotension, impaired cardiac conduction, supraventricular and ventricular arrhythmias, and respiratory depression.

Physostigmine is an antidote for the anticholinergic toxicity, but it should not be used in TCA overdose. Its effects are very short lived, and studies have shown asystole, ventricular arrhythmias, and seizures in patients given this agent. The two most useful agents in treating TCA overdoses are activated charcoal and sodium bicarbonate. Repeated doses of activated charcoal have been shown to be effective in removing many toxins from circulation, including TCAs.

Sodium bicarbonate is extremely important in treating these patients and should be given intravenously until the arterial pH is 7.5. At this point approximately 98% of the tricyclic is protein bound, making it unavailable to tissues and hence limiting its potential for toxicity.

The toxic drug ingested by this patient was fairly clear. When a patient with an overdose of unknown substances presents in an unarousable state, she should be evaluated for the presence of a recognizable toxidrome. Some of the more common and characteristic ones are:

1. *Anticholinergic*—hot flushed skin, tachycardia, dry mucous membranes, mydriasis, altered mental status ("hot as a pistol, red as a beet, dry as a bone, blind as a bat, mad as a hatter").
2. *Cholinergic*—SLUDGE syndrome (Salivation, Lacrimation, Urination, Defecation, Gastrointestinal hypermotility, and Emesis), bradycardia, miosis, wheezing, and respiratory distress.
3. *Sympathomimetic*—hypertension, anxiety, tachycardia, and mydriasis.
4. *Narcotic*—miosis and central nervous system depression, including respiratory depression.
5. *Sedative/Hypnotic*—central nervous system depression, including respiratory depression, with variable pupillary size.

Other poisons may turn up on laboratory analysis. Arterial blood gases clarify the patient's state of oxygenation, and acid base status. Metabolic acidosis is seen in carbon monoxide and cyanide poisoning, and some alcohol poisonings. The serum osmolality will detect the presence of all of the alcohols. The electrolytes will detect an anion gap. Acetaminophen levels must be measured specifically since this drug cannot be detected by clinical or other laboratory means.

REFERENCES

Textbook   Rosen. Pp. 12–14, 1835–1844 (suicide), 2087–2098 (TCA).

Review Article Frommer, D. A., et al. Tricyclic antidepressant overdose: A re-
                    view. *J.A.M.A.* 1987;257:521–526.

Additional   Pentel, P. Asystole complicating physostigmine treatment of tri-
References   cyclic antidepressant overdose. *Ann. Emerg. Med.* 1980;9:
                    588–590.

                    Foulke, G. E. Tricyclic antidepressant overdose. *Am. J. Emerg.
                    Med.* 1986;4:496–500.

                    Wolfe, T. R., Caravati, E. M., and Rollins, D. E. Terminal 40m
                    sec frontal plane QRS axis as a marker for tricyclic anti-
                    depressant overdose. *Ann. Emerg. Med.* 1989;18:348–351.

                    Weissberg, M. P., and Suskauer, S. H. The suicide crisis: Pre-
                    venting the final act. *Emerg. Med. Rep.* 1986;6:105–112.

Case 78 Acting Weird

A distraught mother called her family physician because her 18-year-old daughter was acting strangely. She said that her daughter thought everything was funny and at the same time could not remember anything. At first the mother thought this was a part of an adolescent mood swing, but a few hours after the onset of this behavior, she decided to have the young woman checked. Since it was after office hours, the family doctor asked her to bring the daughter to the emergency department and explained that he would examine her there.

On arrival at the ED, the girl was indeed acting unusually even for an adolescent. She thought that everything was funny, and laughed in response to being questioned. When asked how old she was, she stated it was summer. Her past history was unremarkable, but her mother remembered that the girl had a "cold" several weeks before. Physical examination was completely normal except for the mental status examination. The girl was not oriented to time or place. She was unable, or unwilling, to count backward from 100 by sevens, to interpret proverbs, or to respond to questions about how she was feeling. A complete blood count, routine blood chemistries, and a toxicology screen were drawn and sent to the lab for analysis. A lumbar puncture was performed. All these tests were negative. A neurologic consultant called into the case suggested liver function studies be done to test for the presence of a hepatic encephalopathy. Liver enzymes were elevated as was a serum ammonia level. The patient was transferred by helicopter to a tertiary care center where a diagnosis of Reye's syndrome was made. She recovered with only a mild memory deficit.

What is Reye's syndrome?

What is the hallmark of an acute metabolic encephalopathy?

What is the role of the family doctor in the ED?

DISCUSSION   Reye's syndrome is a form of hepatic encephalopathy associated with viral illnesses, most commonly varicella and influenza
B. This syndrome is strongly associated with aspirin use during
the viral illness. The syndrome is most common in young children, but can also be seen in adolescents and young adults.
The oldest reported case was 63 years old. The initial symptoms are usually vomiting and altered behavior progressing to
stupor and coma. In severe cases there is increased intracranial
pressure. Treatment is supportive, and with good intensive care
the prognosis is usually good. Residual neurologic sequelae are
common but mild. The diagnosis is made in patients with an
acute encephalopathy who have elevated liver function tests
and an otherwise negative workup.

   This patient presented with an acute alteration of her mental
status. A common pitfall in the assessment of these patients is
the assumption that because the patient is alert and just acting
"weird," she probably has an acute psychosis or is under the
influence of drugs. Delirium, an agitated and confused state, is
the hallmark of the patient with an acute organic brain syndrome. To assess brain function, the physician must make a
careful neurologic and mental status examination. A few simple
questions will elicit indication of the more urgent problems:
Does the patient respond to me? Is she awake? Does she know
where she is, how far she is from her home, what day it is, and
about what time of the day it is? Is she responding appropriately
to my presence, or is she struggling with and hostile to someone who is here to help her? If she is confused, hostile, or
asleep and not easily roused to full alertness, then she may
have a life-threatening emergency.

   The immediate workup of the patient with acute organic
brain syndrome includes a complete blood count, glucose, urea
nitrogen, electrolytes, serum osmolarity, and arterial blood
gases. These can be followed by chest x-ray, EKG, CT scan of
the brain, and lumbar puncture. A toxicologic screen may be
helpful later in the patient's course but is rarely available in the
immediate treatment phase. If all these are negative, one must
look for even more unusual causes.

   Physicians in the community will often bring their patients to
the ED for an evaluation after hours. In some cases the patient
evaluation will be done in the ED by the family physician. This
is quite appropriate since he or she knows the patient well. The
emergency physician may function as an informal consultant in
this setting. More often the patient is instructed to come to the
ED for an evaluation by the ED staff. The family physician will

usually call ahead and notify the ED physician of the patient's arrival and discuss the patient's past medical history and current situation with the ED physician. In this setting, as in others, two heads are often better than one.

REFERENCES
Textbook   Tintinalli. Pp. 450–453.

Review Article   Lovejoy, F. H., et al. Clinical staging and Reye syndrome. *Am. J. Dis. Child.* 1974;128:36–41.

Additional   Reye, R. D. K., Morgan, G., and Baral J. Encephalopathy and
References   fatty degeneration of the viscera: A disease entity in child-hood. *Lancet* 1963;2:749–752.

                           Starko, K. M., et al. Reye's syndrome and salicylate use. *Pediatrics* 1980;66:859–864.

Case **79** Diarrhea

A 26-year-old man arrived in the emergency department complaining of diarrhea and crampy abdominal pain. The illness had begun suddenly three days earlier and was accompanied by two episodes of vomiting, slight nausea, and anorexia. He complained of eight to ten watery, foul-smelling bowel movements daily and said that he had to get up several times at night. That day he felt a bit weak and light-headed, especially when he rose quickly. His girlfriend had similar complaints, and although her symptoms were not as severe, they had been present for about ten days. His past medical history was unremarkable, he was taking no medications, and he had no allergies. There was an epidemic of giardiasis in his town.

On examination he appeared in no distress and was afebrile with a supine blood pressure of 120/76, pulse of 84, and respiratory rate of 20. Abdominal examination showed slight tenderness in the periumbilical area and slightly increased bowel sounds. Rectal examination was nontender but the stool was trace positive for occult blood. When he stood up, his blood pressure dropped to 104/64 and his pulse went to 112.

He was given 2 liters of normal saline intravenously over the next two hours. He was also given an injection of dimenhydrinate (Dramamine). Following this he was drowsy but otherwise felt better. When he stood up, he no longer had a drop in blood pressure. A spun hematocrit was 43 initially and dropped to 40 after hydration. A stool sample was obtained for ova and parasites, and he was discharged with a prescription for oral metronidazole and a warning to avoid alcohol while taking that medication. He was to take only clear liquids for the first twenty-four hours and take Kaopectate for the diarrhea. It was also recommended that his girlfriend have a stool sample sent for ova and parasites.

What are the common causes of acute diarrhea?

How should diarrhea be worked up in the ED?

How should dehydration be treated in the ED?

263

DISCUSSION   Giardiasis is not the most common cause of acute infectious diarrhea, but it appears in local epidemic outbreaks. The classic presentation of *Giardia lamblia* infection includes crampy abdominal pain with watery, foul-smelling diarrhea. Nausea and vomiting are occasionally found but are not the prominent symptoms. Diagnosis by stool examination for ova and parasites is fairly accurate in the acute phase, but less accurate as the infection becomes chronic.

The most common causes of acute diarrhea in adults are food poisoning and viral gastroenteritis. Food poisoning, usually caused by staphylococcal toxin, occurs within four hours of ingestion of spoiled food. Abdominal pain, vomiting, and diarrhea are usually severe, but the illness is self-limiting, lasting from eight to twelve hours. Viral gastroenteritis also presents with the triad of abdominal pain, vomiting, and diarrhea but lasts longer. Clustering of cases in the home is common in both diseases. The abdominal examination is variable and frequently changes over the course of a brief observation period in the ED. Acute bacterial enteritis and pseudomembranous enterocolitis are serious but less common causes that must be considered. Bacterial enteritis should be suspected in any patient who appears toxic. Unfortunately, many stool samples may have to be cultured before one gets a diagnostic answer, even in a very sick patient with *Shigella, Campylobacter,* or *Salmonella* enteritis. Pseudomembranous enterocolitis is suspected in any patient who was recently on antibiotics. One looks for *Clostridium difficile* toxin in the stool sample.

Most physicians are unsure of what laboratory tests to order in the workup on these patients. Too much testing is more common than too little. A complete blood count will not differentiate viral from bacterial causes of diarrhea. Electrolyte panels are seldom helpful in young healthy persons. We check electrolytes only on patients who have had serious vomiting or diarrhea over several days, are infants or elderly, are taking diuretics, or who have remarkably abnormal vital signs. It may help to stain the stool for white cells, a sign of bacterial diarrhea which is rarely seen in food poisoning or viral gastroenteritis.

An important examination in any patient with severe diarrhea is to check the vital signs for orthostatic changes. No one is exactly sure what pressure change, on rising from supine to standing, is "significant." Some emergency medicine experts accept a drop of 20 mm Hg in the systolic pressure or a rise of 20 beats per minute in the pulse as suggestive of significant dehydration. We try to estimate the "mean" arterial pressure by adding one-third of the pulse pressure to the diastolic reading. We consider a drop of 10 mm Hg of the mean pressure to be a worrisome fall and 20 mm Hg as quite likely to cause serious symptoms.

When the dehydration is thought to be significant, we treat these patients with intravenous 5% dextrose/0.5 normal saline, and most of them feel better after a liter is given. Medications to stop the vomiting and decrease gastrointestinal hypermotility include dimenhydrinate and prochlorperazine (Compazine). The latter will rarely produce acute dystonic reactions but may worsen hypotension. Diarrhea should not be treated with opiates or other potent antidiarrheal agents since these can increase mucosal invasion in bacterial diarrhea. Antibiotics are usually reserved for the cases of *Shigella* or *Campylobacter*.

Oral rehydration is begun with clear liquids (water, flat ginger ale or other clear sodas, Jello, and clear broth) and advanced gradually to a BRAT (Bananas, Rice or rice cereal, Applesauce, and dry Toast) diet when the vomiting has ceased. We recommend no dairy products for a week after the diarrhea ceases since there is frequently some residual lactose intolerance.

Infants and young children who dehydrate with diarrhea can do so more quickly than adults, due to their smaller fluid reserves. Children who have dry mucous membranes and a somewhat less than usual volume of dark-colored urine are clinically judged to be 5% dehydrated and need volume replacement. Those with lethargy, shrunken fontanelles, tenting of the skin, parched mucous membranes, and little or no urine output are estimated to be 10% or more clinically dehydrated and require intravenous hydration. We usually begin with a bolus of 10 to 20 ml per kg of 5% dextrose/1/3 normal saline over the first hour, while laboratory studies are pending.

REFERENCES

Textbook   Rosen. Pp. 1479–1523, 2259–2270.

Review Article   Wolfe, M. S. Current concepts in parasitology: Giardiasis. *N. Engl. J. Med.* 1978;298:6.

Additional   Bishop, W. P., and Ulshen, M. H. Bacterial gastroenteritis. *Pedi-*
References   *atr. Clin. North Am.* 1988;35:69–88.

                      Mitchell, J. E., and Skelton, M. M. Diarrheal infections. *Am. Fam. Physician* 1988;37:195–207.

American Academy of Pediatrics Committee on Nutrition. Use of oral fluid therapy and posttreatment feeding following enteritis in children in a developed country. *Pediatrics* 1985; 75:358–360.

Case 80 Syncope

A woman was brought to the emergency department by ambulance after she fainted at home. She had been standing at the sink, helping her daughter dry the dinner dishes, when she slumped to the floor and was unconscious for a minute or two. There were no seizure movements and no incontinence, and she was feeling much better when the paramedics arrived.

On arrival at the ED, she said that she was "as well as one could be for 76 years." She denied smoking or drinking and said that she took only the Aldomet and digoxin her physician prescribed. She had never fainted before and had been feeling well earlier in the day. The examining doctor found that she had a pulse of 74 and a blood pressure of 134/80. He found nothing remarkable in his examination of her heart, lungs, and abdomen and no lateralizing neurologic findings.

Since it was her first faint, the doctor obtained some laboratory studies. A chest x-ray showed slightly increased interstitial markings. A cardiogram showed sinus rhythm with normal intervals but demonstrated ST sagging and T-wave flattening across the precordium. Her electrolytes and BUN were normal as were her complete blood count and urinalysis. Because of the T-wave abnormalities, the doctor wondered about a pulmonary embolism and obtained an emergency perfusion-ventilation lung scan that was interpreted by the radiologist on call as "low probability of pulmonary embolism, although not entirely normal."

The patient insisted that she felt well and wanted to go home. Accordingly, she was discharged to be taken home by her daughter, who was much reassured by all the normal tests but a little worried about the T waves and the "not quite normal lung scan."

The next day, while getting dressed to go shopping, the patient fainted again. This time she woke unattended on the floor. She called her daughter and asked to be taken to her usual doctor. He found her blood pressure acceptable in the supine or seated position but 80/50 when she stood up. He gave her a liter of saline intravenously in his office, recommended drinking

267

more water and salting her food liberally for a few days and stopped her alpha-methyl dopa. She did well with his therapy.

The following week she received a bill for $780 for the ED treatment.

What are the essentials of an ED evaluation for fainting?

What was left out in this case?

DISCUSSION   Fainting is common. Our first task is to distinguish a seizure from a faint and then to look for causes of syncope. In an elderly woman, one must worry about causes for decreased brain blood flow, most of which are to be found in the heart and blood vessels rather than in the brain. Surely a careful cardiovascular examination is necessary, and nothing can replace careful vital signs, including an observation of the effect of sitting up and then standing. This patient was examined entirely in the supine position. Even her history cried out for a standing evaluation since she was standing when she fainted.

Many drugs may cause postural drops in blood pressure, usually those that are direct vasodilators (e.g., nitrates, calcium channel blockers, phenothiazines, narcotics, and hydralazine and other alpha blockers), or diuretics, or those that prevent the usual cardiac response to hypotension (beta blockers.) Of course any drug used to decrease blood pressure may do its job too well and produce hypotension.

If you are unable to document postural hypotension, your attention should turn to cardiac arrhythmias as the next most common cause of syncope in the elderly. Bradycardias, heart block, and rapid tachycardias can all cause syncope. In fact, since the first visit to the ED failed to find a clear cause for her syncope, it would have been reasonable to admit her to the hospital and place her on a cardiac monitor. An arrhythmia may have been missed.

It is embarrassing when a simple maneuver like taking the blood pressure is found to be more useful than all the technology we are so proud of. Postural blood pressure readings cost considerably less than this patient's visit to our ED. She had reason to be puzzled and even distressed about our failure to diagnose her problem.

REFERENCES
Textbook   Rosen. Pp. 1790–1798.

Review Article Linzer, M. Syncope. *South. Med. J.* 1987;80:545–553.

Additional   Silverstein, M. D., et al. Patients with syncope admitted to med-
Reference   ical intensive care units. *J.A.M.A.* 1982;248:1185–1189.

Case 81 Respiratory Infection

A 26-year-old man came to the emergency department complaining of a cold. He thought that a shot of penicillin would clear him up. He claimed a cough productive of about one shotglass (2 ounces) of green-yellow sputum daily for the past week. The cough was associated with a ripping substernal pain that he said felt like he was "coming apart with the cough." He smoked about one-and-a-half packs of cigarettes a day but commented that he seldom finished a cigarette and that his friends bummed many cigarettes from him, contributing to that total. In describing his smoking, he said that he smoked "not too much." He also commented on a stuffy head but denied earache, ear drainage, or severe headaches. He noted mild hoarseness. He thought that shortness of breath was not a problem but that recently any activity was causing coughing spells that were hard to stop. Deep breathing also would provoke such a spell, and the coughing frequently led to retching. He denied any drug allergies.

On physical exam, the patient had a temperature of 37.5°C orally, a respiratory rate of 18, a pulse of 94, and a blood pressure of 130/84 in the right arm when seated. His pharynx was a bit red; his tympanic membranes were normal. He had no tenderness over the maxillary sinuses or under the supraorbital ridge. His voice was slightly rough, and he sniffled frequently. As he took a deep breath, a vibratory sensation was palpable bilaterally over the middle ribs laterally. With a stethoscope, coarse rhonchi were audible. When asked to cough, he produced a few milliliters of yellow sputum.

What is a "cold"?

What does this patient have?

How would you treat this patient?

DISCUSSION The popular term *cold* has no exact medical significance but usually is equated with a viral upper respiratory infection. "Upper respiratory" is usually taken to mean bronchi and above, leaving the bronchioles and lungs to the "lower respiratory" system. Thus, upper respiratory symptoms include headache, earache, ear drainage, tinnitus, rhinorrhea, stuffy head, sore throat, pain on swallowing, swollen cervical nodes, loss of voice, and cough. Lower respiratory symptoms are chiefly three: cough, shortness of breath, and chest pain. Upper respiratory infections are either viral or bacterial. Viral upper respiratory infections (URIs) include mononucleosis. In adults, penicillin generally is good therapy if a strep throat is diagnosed, otherwise use ampicillin since other organisms such as haemophilus and neisseria species are often seen as well.

Severe hoarseness to the point of aphonia or severe dysphagia, or both, may be the presentation of acute epiglottitis in an adult. This is a rare bacterial upper respiratory infection and deserves hospitalization and immediate ENT consultation. To try to visualize the posterior pharynx or epiglottis in an epiglottitis patient can be a fatal error if one is not prepared with equipment at hand to do an emergency intubation or cricothyrotomy.

In this patient a chest x-ray may reveal bronchopneumonia but will probably be normal. The diagnosis is bronchitis, and the etiology may be either viral or bacterial. With yellow or green sputum we usually treat bronchitis with an antibiotic and currently pick ampicillin, erythromycin, or trimethoprim/sulfamethoxazole as a first choice.

At least as important, the patient should be told to stop smoking during this illness (and preferably thereafter). He should be encouraged to drink copious amounts of nonalcoholic fluids and to obtain some means of inhaling a high-humidity atmosphere to aid him in bringing up sputum. Many patients will request cough medicines, but the patient with a productive cough or fever should not usually be given powerful cough suppressants such as codeine: He needs his cough to drain the purulent secretions. If given at all, codeine should be limited to nighttime use to allow sleep or used only occasionally to minimize prolonged, painful coughing fits.

REFERENCES
Textbook Rosen. Pp. 1097–1101.

Review Article   Baker, L. R., et al. Respiratory Infections. *Principles of Ambulatory Care Medicine,* 2nd edition. Baltimore, Williams & Wilkins, 1986. Pp. 357–359.

Additional   Dunway, J., and Reinhardt, R. Clinical features and treatments
Reference   of acute bronchitis. *J. Fam. Pract.* 1984;18:719–722.

Case 82 Sudden Shoulder Pain

A 34-year-old physician came to the emergency department by private car. He arrived walking bent over with his left arm held before him flexed at the elbow. He said that he was having terrible pain in his left shoulder and that it had begun fifteen minutes earlier, just after he had thrown a 50-pound bag of wood chips in his backyard. This was the sixth time he had suffered such an episode.

On examination, once the patient's shirt was removed, he seemed in much distress and was somewhat pale and sweaty. His right shoulder curvature was more rounded than the left, and there was a bulge anteriorly on the left side. He could not move his upper arm and complained much of pain.

What is the diagnosis in this case?

Should x-rays be taken?

What can you do to relieve this patient?

DISCUSSION   This patient has a recurring anterior shoulder dislocation. He probably should have a shoulder capsule reconstruction to avoid further recurrences. At the present time, the object is to reduce his dislocation. Although fractures are seldom true emergencies, dislocations more often are, since nerve and vascular supplies may be damaged. A distal neurovascular examination should be done before and after reduction looking for decreased sensation, diminished pulses, or delayed capillary refill. (Capillary refill is delayed if it takes longer for the normal color to return than for the examiner to say "capillary refill" to himself.) Your patient will thank you for being brisk in your examination. His priority is for you to reduce the dislocation as soon as possible.

We commonly see dislocated fingers, toes, shoulders, patellas, and hips. Dislocations of the hip often are difficult to reduce, whereas dislocations of fingers and toes can usually be easily reduced in the ED. One very easily reduced subluxation is the "nursemaid's elbow"—the radial head subluxation of childhood. It typically occurs when a walking child's arm is forcibly pulled, often by the parent. Reduction can be performed by supination and flexion of the involved elbow and is often performed by the x-ray technician when positioning the child to have the elbow x-rayed. A palpable pop indicates reduction and the child will begin to use the arm normally within a short observation time.

Although we always x-ray a dislocation when it is a first-time event, we sometimes do not wait to obtain x-rays on repeat cases. The likelihood of a fracture-dislocation being present is very low in this case.

For anterior shoulder dislocation such as this case, we generally use intravenous diazepam (Valium) and 5 to 10 mg of morphine for analgesia and then attempt to reduce the shoulder dislocation. This patient was given 10 mg of Valium intravenously. Then, a sheet about his torso was pulled to the right, a large towel about his upper arm pulled to the left, and gentle manipulation of the arm flexed at the elbow led to relocation of the shoulder. A number of other methods achieve the same results.

Once a dislocation is reduced, the pain diminishes radically, and any analgesia present will have much more effect. The patient often goes to sleep, and we have to beware of a respiratory arrest if a large dose of analgesic was given.

Prior to discharge, the dislocated joint must be fully immobilized. In shoulder dislocations we use a "sling and swathe" (a sling strapped to the torso).

REFERENCES
Textbook   Rosen. Pp. 740–746.

Review Article   Lambert, W., and Egherman, W. Emergency diagnosis and
                      management of common shoulder injuries. *Emerg. Med. Rep.*
                      1987;8:185–192.

Additional   Boger, D., Sipsui, J. M., and Anderson, J. New traction devices
References   to aid reduction of shoulder dislocations. *Ann. Emerg. Med.*
                      1984;13:423–425.

                      Cone, R. O., and Resnicks, D. Traumatic disorders of the shoul-
                      der. *J.A.M.A.* 1984;252:540–543.

Case 83 Hit by a Car

A 48-year-old man was struck by a fast-moving automobile. Paramedics found him to be confused with a blood pressure of 90/50 mm Hg. He was rapidly immobilized on a long board and transported to the emergency department. On arrival he was diaphoretic and cool with a blood pressure of 70/50, pulse of 120, and respiratory rate of 40.

His breath sounds were equal and clear, and his abdomen was distended and mildly tender. His pelvis was tender on compression of both the iliac crests and pubic symphysis. Blood was present at the urethral meatus, and the rectal exam revealed a "high riding" prostate. His right thigh was swollen and his left leg deformed with the foot rotated externally. His right upper arm was swollen and bruised, but there was no evidence of neurovascular compromise.

Intravenous access was obtained for fluid resuscitation and x-ray examination initiated. Cervical spine and chest x-rays were normal. The pelvic film showed a diastasis (separation) of the pubic symphysis. Extremity films showed a right femur fracture, comminuted left tibia and fibula fractures, and a right humerus fracture. Because of the possibility of urethral injury, a retrograde urethrogram was performed that showed a posterior urethral rupture. He was taken to the operating room for further fluid resuscitation, pelvic fracture stabilization, and repair of his urethral injury.

Where exactly should paramedics take patients like this?

What are priorities in pelvic fractures?

DISCUSSION   Patients with multiple trauma and hypotension, coma, or respiratory failure should be transferred to a regional trauma center as soon as possible. With long transport times, these patients may be stabilized at a nearby hospital and subsequently transferred to a designated trauma center. Studies have shown that bypassing general hospitals and taking such patients directly to a trauma center saves lives. Regional prehospital protocols usually define which patients require trauma center care.

Pelvic fractures usually involve multiple disruptions of the pelvic ring. A single fracture of the pelvic ring, like a single crack in a Lifesavers candy, is almost impossible. Multiple or displaced fractures are often unstable. Massive and fatal hemorrhage can occur from pelvic veins, arterial disruption, and the fracture site itself, which has a generous blood supply. MAST pants, when used in this setting, help to stabilize the fractures as well as maintain the blood pressure. Be careful when deflating them because too-rapid deflation can cause a precipitous drop in the blood pressure of an otherwise stable-appearing patient.

As always, aggressive fluid resuscitation is required if shock is present. Additional venous access may be required. When the vital signs reveal shock, an initial fluid bolus of 20 ml per kg (or 10 ml per pound) is appropriate.

When the pelvis is fractured, rectal, ureteral, and bladder injuries may be found. Blood at the urethral meatus, an inability to void, and high-riding prostate on rectal exam are cardinal signs of urethral injury. Generally a Foley catheter should not be placed in these patients until a retrograde urethrogram is performed. An IVP to rule out higher injury usually follows. The mortality rate for patients with open pelvic fractures is over 50% due to hemorrhage, infection, and associated injury.

REFERENCES
Textbook   Rosen. Pp. 817–831.

Review Article Snyder, H. Blunt pelvic trauma. *Am. J. Emerg. Med.* 1988;6:618–627.

Additional   Schneider, P. A., Mitchell, J. M., and Allison, E. J. The use of
References   military antishock trousers in trauma—a reevaluation. *J. Emerg. Med.* 1989;7:497–500.

Civil, I. D., et al. Routine pelvic radiography and severe blunt trauma: Is it necessary? *Ann. Emerg. Med.* 1988;17:488–490.

Trunkey, D. D. Management of pelvic fractures in blunt trauma injury. *J. Trauma* 1974;14:912–923.

Case 84 Kicked in the Groin

A 15-year-old boy came to the emergency department complaining of abdominal pain and nausea that had begun suddenly four hours before. He said that his right testicle was swollen and that "something like this" had happened in the past, but went away spontaneously. Today he had played football and had been kicked in the groin. He had been sexually active for almost a year but never had any sexually transmitted diseases, urethral discharge, or pain on urinating.

On physical examination he was noted to be an athletic adolescent male in marked distress. His temperature was 100°F, pulse 120, respiratory rate 18, and blood pressure 110/80. His abdomen was normal, but his scrotum was red and warm, with a tender and swollen right testicle.

His white blood cell count was 10,000 per mm³, and his urinalysis showed 5 white cells per high-power field.

What is the diagnosis?

What diagnostic studies might be helpful?

Why is a prompt diagnosis so important?

DISCUSSION   In this case the priority diagnosis is testicular torsion. It is not
the most common cause of a swollen testicle, but it is the most
urgent. Although the peak incidence is in adolescence, it can be
seen in adults, premature infants, and the elderly as well. Unde-
scended testes have a tenfold increased incidence of torsion.

With a "bell clapper" deformity, the tunica vaginalis is capac-
ious and has no posterior attachment. This allows the testicle to
twist, compressing vessels and causing ischemia. The degree of
testicular atrophy that follows torsion is proportional to the degree and duration of the torsion, so early diagnosis is important.
If the diagnosis is made within six hours of the onset of symptoms, the salvage rate approaches 100%. In another six hours,
only 20% of testes can be saved.

The classic presentation consists of the sudden onset of severe unrelenting pain that may be referred to the inguinal or
abdominal region. In the classic description, the twisted testicle
sits high and the epididymis is in an abnormal position. The
scrotum is red and edematous, and often a reactive hydrocele
has formed obscuring the testicle. These patients rarely tolerate
a careful examination because of severe pain. It was once
thought that if elevation of the testicle gave pain relief, then
epididymitis was more likely than torsion. This feature, Prehn's
sign, is now known to be unreliable. About a fifth of patients
with torsion have fever and a third have pyuria.

In the differential diagnosis, one must consider acute epididymitis, orchitis, and torsion of the appendix testis. Testicular
cancer, which also tends to occur in young patients, may present with a swollen, red scrotum, although *usually* it is a painless condition.

Doppler flow studies are a quick and easy bedside test. If
flow is not detected on the tender side, then torsion is likely.
Unfortunately, detection of flow does not rule out torsion as
increased scrotal flow may mimic testicular blood flow.

The diagnosis of testicular torsion is made correctly on clinical grounds only 50% of the time. Radioactive technetium
scanning is somewhat more accurate than Doppler and is often
used in equivocal cases. Unfortunately both Doppler and nucle-
ar studies have false-positives and false-negatives. To obtain
definitive diagnosis of the swollen, tender testicle, surgical exploration is most reliable. In adolescent and prepubertal boys
where there is significant doubt about the diagnosis, surgical
exploration should be undertaken. While the operating room is
being prepared, manual detorsion may be attempted. Even if
this is successful, an operation including exploration and surgi-

cal fixation of both testes within the scrotum (orchiopexy) is still mandatory, since recurrence is common.

REFERENCES
Textbook   Rosen. Pp. 1556–1560.

Review Article   Edelsberg, J. S., and Surhy, S. The acute scrotum. *Emerg. Med. Clin. North Am.* 1988;6:521–548.

Additional   Lindsey, D., and Stanisic, T. H. Diagnosis and management of
References   testicular torsion: Pitfalls and perils. *Am. J. Emerg. Med.* 1988;6:42–46.

                      Cattolica, A. V. Preoperative manual detorsion of the torsed spermatic cord. *J. Urol.* 1985;133:803–805.

Case 85 Child with a Barking Cough

A 4-year-old boy was brought to the emergency department at midnight because of difficulty breathing. He had had a low-grade fever and nasal congestion all day and began having noisy breathing and a barking cough in the middle of the night. The parents described the noise on inspiration to their pediatrician over the phone and he requested them to bring the child right to the ED for examination.

The child appeared to be in no acute distress and was breathing more comfortably than at home. His temperature was 103.6°F, and he had frequent bouts of a barking cough. Further examination showed no abnormalities except a slightly red throat, and his parents were told to give him acetaminophen and use a cool mist humidifier at his bedside at home.

Several hours later they returned to the ED because the child began having more trouble breathing and could not lie down. The boy was sitting on the stretcher and was noted by a nurse to be drooling. His temperature was then 104.2°F. The pediatric resident seemed annoyed over having been wakened from sleep to see the child again. He asked the child to open his mouth, and when the child opened it only a small amount, the resident became angry, asked a nurse to restrain him, and placed a tongue blade in the mouth to visualize the tonsils better.

The child had a sudden respiratory arrest. Attempts were made to intubate him, but a large, red, swollen epiglottis prevented this, and after about five to six minutes (since there was a great deal of confusion, no one kept track of the time), a surgeon was called to perform an emergency tracheostomy. The airway was finally established, and a stable cardiac rhythm returned, but the child never regained consciousness and was pronounced brain dead several days later.

What is croup and when should the suspicion of epiglottitis be raised?

What is the correct treatment of epiglottitis in a child?

DISCUSSION   Acute epiglottitis in a child is an immediately life-threatening emergency. This case occurred seventeen years ago, and along with many other similar cases has led to the use of strict protocols for the treatment of this disease. Whenever a child with a clinical picture of acute epiglottitis (high fever, inspiratory stridor, drooling, and sitting forward unwilling to speak or move) presents to our ED, a predetermined plan is set in motion. The operating room is immediately readied and an anesthesiologist and otolaryngologist are called. A "double setup" is prepared and brought to the bedside so the staff has the equipment at hand to endotracheally intubate or, if necessary, perform a cricothyrotomy. The child is made as comfortable as possible and is given humidified oxygen. No blood is drawn or intravenous line established at this point, although an intravenous antibiotic for presumed *Haemophilus* epiglottitis will be begun once the airway is secured. If he begins to tire or obstruct before the team is assembled, ventilations may be assisted with a bag-valve-mask apparatus. Once in the operating room, orotracheal intubation is attempted under inhalational anesthesia. If this fails, an emergency cricothyrotomy or tracheostomy is performed. This protocol has reduced the mortality for this disease.

Croup is usually a viral infection causing swelling of the subglottic area and is not as life-threatening as epiglottitis. The child is usually between the ages of 6 months and 3 years—somewhat younger than the usual epiglottitis patient—although there is so much overlap that age alone is not a reliable way to differentiate one from the other. In croup, the "croupy" (honking, barking) cough is usually preceded by an upper respiratory infection. Typically, the illness progresses slowly over days, as opposed to the more rapid progression over a single day typical of epiglottitis. The characteristic barking cough sound is unmistakable. Most children improve after they are taken into a steamy shower, or while being driven to the ED. If the child arrives in severe respiratory distress, immediate treatment with racemic epinephrine given by a small-volume nebulizer may be lifesaving. The relief, however, is short lived and frequently a rebound phenomenon occurs that results in stridor as bad or worse than the original condition. Any child treated with epinephrine should be hospitalized to get repeated treatments until better. Most children need only humidified air for treatment and can be discharged to their home. If there is still a question of epiglottitis after the child has been clinically evaluated, a good-quality soft tissue lateral neck x-ray can differentiate croup from epiglottitis in most cases.

REFERENCES
Textbook   Fleisher. Pp. 433–438.

Review Article   Hen, J. Current management of upper airway obstruction. *Pe-diatr. Ann.* 1986;15:274–294.

Additional   Hodge, K. M., and Ganzel, T. M. Diagnostic and therapeutic
References   efficiency in croup and epiglottitis. *Laryngoscope* 1987;97:
                        621–625.

                        Singer, J. I., and McCabe, J. B. Epiglottitis at the extremes of
                        age. *Am. J. Emerg. Med.* 1988;6:228–231.

                        Willis, R. J., and Roland, T. W. The early management of acute
                        epiglottitis: A survey of current practice. *J. Emerg. Med.*
                        1984;2:13–16.

                        Losek, J. D., et al. Epiglottitis: Comparison of signs and symp-
                        toms in children less than two years old and older. *Ann.
                        Emerg. Med.* 1990;19:55–59.

Case 86 Motorcycle Accident

A 20-year-old was riding his motorcycle too fast on a country road when he lost control and the bike fell over. He and the bike slid down the road 75 feet and smashed into a guard rail. The noise was heard by nearby neighbors, who soon called an ambulance. The volunteers arrived about fifteen minutes later, and since they had little training they provided the patient with a "scoop and run" transport that involved little medical care but did get him to the hospital promptly. On arrival, he was awake and screaming, "I am all right . . . Get me out of here . . . I can't breathe . . . Get me out of here . . . I can't breathe." He had no apparent injury other than a bleeding cut over his eyebrow. Several minutes were spent trying to coax him to stay on the hospital stretcher and trying to obtain a blood pressure reading despite his lack of cooperation. He had no obvious chest injury, but auscultation of his lungs was difficult since he was still talking loudly and thrashing about. Shortly thereafter, the staff noticed that he was more cooperative with their attempts to start intravenous lines—in fact, he was soon not moving at all. Vital signs were noted to be absent, and cardiopulmonary resuscitation was begun. During the resuscitation, a chest x-ray was taken. After about twenty minutes of unsuccessful attempts at resuscitation, "the code was called" and the man pronounced dead. Just then the x-ray technician returned with the chest film. It showed a tension pneumothorax.

What are the priorities in the initial evaluation of a multiple-trauma patient?

DISCUSSION   This young man died in the hands of three physicians who were
diligently working to save his life. These three, a surgeon, an
emergency physician, and an anesthesiologist all missed the
diagnosis of an easily treatable and reversible condition. No one
diagnosed a tension pneumothorax because no one looked for
it. The patient probably would have been saved if an 18-gauge
needle had been poked through his chest wall in the second
interspace at the midclavicular line.

Preventable trauma deaths are surprisingly common: We estimate thousands of cases per year in the United States alone.
There is a natural tendency on the part of the physician to
make a treatment and stabilization plan for the patient based on
the type of accident. With an infinite number of accident sce-
narios, plans for patient care could be quite varied, and this
variation can lead to oversight. A better approach stresses a
standardized approach to the trauma patient, regardless of the
mechanism of injury. The American College of Surgeons' Advanced Trauma Life Support course recommends four steps: a
primary survey, including the ABCs; a primary resuscitation
phase, including initial interventions such as oxygen, intravenous fluids, and treatment of immediately life-threatening injuries; a secondary survey, including a head-to-toe physical examination; and then definitive care.

A mnemonic for the necessary actions in the first few minutes
of care is A, B, C, Strip, Hemorrhage, Shock, Splint Major
Fractures, Survey.

A—Airway	If the patient is talking clearly, the airway is ade-quate, at least at that moment.
B—Breathing	We must not only look for adequate ventilation, but consider the three major injuries that can rapidly lead to patient deterioration: tension pneumotho-rax, sucking chest wound, and flail chest.
C—Circulation	Does the patient have an adequate pulse and blood pressure?
Strip	You cannot adequately evaluate a multiple-trauma patient who has his clothes on.
Hemorrhage	You do not have to stop every little cut from bleed-ing, but you do need to stem life-threatening hem-orrhage rapidly. You should be able to stop bleeding from any blood vessel in the body with one or two well-placed fingers; although with some vessels, such as the aorta, getting your fin-gers in the right place is difficult.

Shock	At least two large-bore intravenous lines are needed. 18-gauge is considered small bore in this setting.
Splint Major Fractures	Not every broken finger needs to be fixed at this time, but major unstable long bone fractures need to be immobilized early. Do not waste time here, but quick stabilization will prevent further soft tissue injury and may decrease the incidence of acute respiratory distress syndrome from "fat embolism."
Survey	Two-minute head-to-toe initial survey.

During the first five minutes of care of a multiple-trauma patient, there is always time to consider what should be done next.

And remember: It is very hard to check vital signs too often.

REFERENCES

Textbook   Rosen. Pp. 473–518.

Review   American College of Surgeons' Committee on Trauma. *Advanced Trauma Life Support Program.* Chicago, American College of Surgeons, 1989.

Additional   Mattox, K. L., et al. Thoracic trauma. *Surg. Clin. North Am.*
References   1986;69:1–173.

Kulshrestha, P., et al. Chest injuries: A clinical and autopsy profile. *J. Trauma* 1988;28:844–847.

Carrero, R., and Wayne, M. Chest trauma. *Emerg. Med. Clin. North Am.* 1989;7:389–418.

Case 87 Child with Small Toys

A 3-year-old boy was brought in by his mother because of a fever and drainage from his nose. He had been seen two days before by his pediatrician because of the runny nose, was thought to have a viral upper respiratory infection, and was treated with a decongestant. His nasal drainage became worse and the fever developed. His past history was unremarkable.

When seen in the emergency department, he had a temperature of 102.6°F but was cheerful and played with his mother when not annoyed by our examination. His head and neck were normal except for congestion of the right naris with a large amount of purulent discharge. This was vigorously suctioned, and a small wooden bead was seen inside the nose. The bead could be removed only with difficulty by the ENT resident who was called to see the child.

The child was discharged after we instructed his mother to use salt water nose drops and to keep him away from small toys.

Two weeks later the same child was back. The mother stated that he was playing when he had a sudden coughing spell and perhaps even turned blue for a few seconds. She reported seeing no small toys in the area. He now seemed fine, and his examination was completely normal. Because aspiration was suspected, a chest x-ray was taken. Since it was normal, the child was sent home and the mother reassured.

The next day, the child awoke with a fever and was returned to the ED. He had been coughing all night, his appetite was poor, and he was not interested in playing.

His temperature then was 102.4°F, his pulse 124 per minute, and respirations 36 per minute. Examination was normal except for his chest, which showed wheezes and rhonchi in the right lower lung field. A repeat chest x-ray showed a right middle lobe infiltrate with atelectasis. The child was admitted.

What types of respiratory foreign bodies can cause problems in children?

When should aspiration be suspected?

DISCUSSION   Small children may place toys or other objects in any orifice of the body. This exploratory behavior is common and usually harmless. For this reason, pediatricians advise that children this age have no toy smaller than their fist. Small beads or beans are commonly placed in the nose or ears, and unilateral drainage from the nose or ear suggests the presence of a foreign body. Removal may be accomplished using an ear curette, suction, or fine forceps. Irrigation with water should not be used when beans or vegetable matter have been inserted because this will cause the object to swell.

Aspirated foreign bodies should be considered to be a medical emergency. If the patient is old enough, he may show the universal signs of a choking victim, which are the inability to speak and a hand held to the throat. For a voiceless child who is turning blue, the Heimlich maneuver, rapid upward thrusts into the midepigastrium, may help. Any person who has "choked" and is still able to speak can also breathe and should be left alone until the object can be removed under direct observation.

A more subtle and common presentation occurred in this child. The typical history of sudden choking or coughing while the child was playing should prompt the physician to suspect a foreign body aspiration. The child may have a new cough and occasionally some blood-tinged sputum, although there may be surprisingly few objective signs in the first day. A chest x-ray should be obtained to look for a radiopaque foreign body or evidence of air trapping. Initial hyperinflation on the affected side (due to a one-way valve effect) with a tracheal shift toward the other side, but no pneumothorax, should be taken as evidence of a retained foreign body. Treatment is bronchoscopy and removal of the foreign body. If the child is left untreated, complications include recurrent pneumonias and atelectasis.

REFERENCES
Textbook   Rosen. Pp. 89–95, 125–126, 951–955.

Review Article Mofenson, H. C., and Greensher, J. Management of the choking child. *Pediatr. Clin. North Am.* 1985;32:183–192.

Additional   Standards and guidelines for cardiopulmonary resuscitation and
References   emergency cardiac care. *J.A.M.A.* 1986;255(Suppl.):2841–3044.

Heimlich, H. J. A life saving maneuver to prevent food-choking. *J.A.M.A.* 1975;234:398–401.

Case 88 Child After a Seizure

A previously healthy 2-year-old boy was brought to the emergency department after a generalized tonic-clonic seizure lasting ten minutes. Following a five-minute postictal period, he appeared well. The child's past medical history, developmental history, and family history were unremarkable and included no history of seizures. The child's mother had noted that he had nasal congestion and diarrhea for two days prior to his ED visit. Examination revealed a happy, playful child, in no distress, with the following vital signs: temperature 102°F rectally, pulse 120, blood pressure 85/50 mm Hg, and 28 respirations per minute. His pupils were equal and reactive. Both tympanic membranes were red and immobile. The pharynx was erythematous, without exudate. No adenopathy was noted and his neck was supple. Further examination revealed clear lungs, a nontender abdomen, and a normal neurologic examination. The child was discharged with a diagnosis of bilateral otitis media and febrile seizure. Treatment was initiated with amoxicillin and acetaminophen.

Should the child have had a lumbar puncture to rule out meningitis?

Can you have bacterial meningitis without meningeal signs?

DISCUSSION   Febrile seizures occur in 2 to 5% of children under 5 years of age. A simple febrile seizure lasts less than fifteen minutes, is generalized, and occurs between 3 months and 5 years of age in an otherwise normal child who is left with no residual focal neurologic deficit. Atypical febrile seizures may last longer, manifest focal seizure activity, result in a focal neurologic deficit during the postictal period, or recur within twenty-four hours. Febrile seizures usually result from a focus of infection detected on physical exam, e.g., pharyngitis or otitis media, and the primary infection may be treated with antipyretics and appropriate antibiotics, if indicated, in an otherwise well-appearing child. If the child appears ill or the febrile seizures are atypical, a more thorough evaluation must be performed to rule out sepsis and meningitis (blood cultures, lumbar puncture, and occasionally CT scanning).

Examination of a febrile child begins with a complete history, including respiratory complaints, gastrointestinal symptoms, rashes, and any changes in the child's appetite or level of activity. The physical exam should add additional information as to the potential source of infection.

In a child younger than 2 years old, fever over 102°F may result from many causes, including pharyngitis, tracheobronchitis, otitis media, pneumonia, cellulitis, osteomyelitis, appendicitis, septic arthritis, or urinary tract infection. The absence of a specific source of infection despite physical examination, chest x-ray, and urinalysis should raise the index of suspicion for sepsis, bacteremia, and meningitis. Although experts differ about what constitutes the appropriate workup for a febrile infant, we think that if no source of infection is found, a blood culture should be obtained in any child younger than 2 years with a temperature over 104°F, sedimentation rate greater than 30 mm per hour, or a white blood cell count over 15,000 because of a high risk of "occult bacteremia." Additionally, a lumbar puncture is indicated in these cases if the infant appears ill.

Meningitis is a devastating disease with high morbidity and mortality unless diagnosed and treated early. Gram-negative rods and group B streptococcus are the major pathogens in neonatal meningitis. After the first month of life, the major pathogens include pneumococcus, *Haemophilus influenzae,* and meningococcus. Meningitis must always be considered in the febrile child who appears ill or lacks a clear focus of infection. Younger children may present with lethargy, irritability, and decreased feeding as the only symptoms. In children under 6 months of age, and particularly in children under 3 months of age, signs of nuchal rigidity may be subtle or absent. Treatment may involve ampicillin and gentamicin (neonatal meningitis) or chloramphenicol. The newer third-generation cephalosporins (e.g., ceftriaxone, cefotaxime) provide excellent coverage and penetrate the cerebrospinal fluid well and are becoming the drug of choice in older children.

Because this child had such a clear source of infection, a history consistent with a simple febrile seizure, and a happy, playful demeanor in the ED, we think deferring the lumbar puncture was appropriate.

REFERENCES
Textbook   Fleisher. Pp. 163–170, 392–393, 419–426.

Review Article   Bettis, D. B., and Ater, S. B. Febrile seizures: Emergency department diagnosis and treatment. *J. Emerg. Med.* 1985;2: 341–348.

Additional   Keroack, M. A. The patient with suspected meningitis. *Emerg.*
References   *Med. Clin. North Am.* 1987;5:807–826.

                      Stutman, H. R., and Marks, M. I. Bacterial meningitis in children: Diagnosis and therapy. *Clin. Pediatr.* 1987;26:428–431.

                      Chessare, J. B., and Berwick, D. M. Variation in clinical practice in the management of febrile seizures. *Pediatr. Emerg. Care* 1985;1:19–21.

Case 89 Abscess

A 24-year-old muscular male presented to the triage desk complaining of a sore arm, fever, and chills. The patient said he was an intravenous drug user and that several days earlier he had been attempting to "shoot" what he thought was a combination of heroin and cocaine. It had not worked, and he thought he missed the vein with at least part of the solution. By the next day, his arm had become warm, sore, and swollen, and this had continued to progress rapidly until he decided to come to the hospital. When he started to get sick, he inquired of his friends who suggested that perhaps the packet he had injected contained Ritalin and not cocaine. The examining physician found a huge fluctuant abscess extending down the lateral side of his arm from the deltoid muscle to the elbow. The patient required an incision and drainage, and it took five full bottles of iodoform gauze packing to fill the cavity.

Is this a "boil"?

How is it treated?

DISCUSSION   An abscess usually begins with a small break in the skin or a superficial skin infection. If caused by staphylococcus, the infection may spread deeper and cause a "boil," a subcutaneous collection of pus surrounded by an area of cellulitis. Although antibiotic therapy will reduce and control the cellulitis around the pus collection, the only effective treatment of an abscess is drainage.

Adequate anesthesia is usually difficult to obtain. One option is to use a field block around the abscess. Lidocaine is injected in a ring surrounding the abscess and then subcutaneously over the area where the incision is to be made. The incision can then be made into the abscess cavity and pus released. A common error in this procedure is not going deep enough into the abscess cavity; there are usually fibrous septae in the cavity when it is large, and these must be broken up either with a clamp or the physician's finger. The cavity should then be packed open with gauze to prevent it from closing and the abscess from reforming. The packing should be removed every two days and replaced with a smaller amount of gauze until the abscess cavity fills in.

Systemic antibiotics are usually not appropriate in the treatment of superficial abscesses but should be used in immunocompromised patients and when there is a large area of cellulitis or ascending lymphangitis associated with the abscess. Cultures of the abscess contents are usually not necessary and should only be taken if the patient is to be placed on antibiotics.

Deep perirectal abscesses, tendon sheath abscesses, and intracavitary abscesses usually require hospitalization and parenteral antibiotics.

Abscesses in drug abusers arise from multiple causes. The needle may be contaminated with bacteria or the drug itself may cause the abscess. This is especially true with sympathomimetics, such as cocaine and amphetamines ("speed"), which produce intense vasoconstriction and cell necrosis at the site of subcutaneous injection. Ritalin is a synthetic amphetamine-like drug with similar properties when injected.

This abscess is unusual in size and shape. One must wonder about its extent and consider unusual bacteria that tend to produce spreading infections that dissect along tissue planes. *Clostridium* species, for example, may be present. Any unusual infection deserves the best help our microbiology lab can give us. We should culture aerobically and anaerobically, and this patient should be hospitalized for observation and intravenous antibiotics. He may be immunosuppressed.

REFERENCES

Textbook   Rosen. Pp. 1004–1009.

Review Article Burney, R. E. Incision and drainage procedures. *Emerg. Med. Clin. North Am.* 1986;4:527–542.

Additional   Meislin, H. W. Pathogenic identification of abscesses and cellu-
References   litus. *Ann. Emerg. Med.* 1986;15:329–332.

Bidernan, P., and Hiatt, J. R. Management of soft-tissue infections of the upper extremity in parenteral drug abusers. *Am. J. Surg.* 1987;154:526–528.

Case 90 Cardiac Arrest

A 55-year-old man developed chest pain while walking to work. When he got to his office, his coworkers noted that he was pale and diaphoretic and called the paramedics through the fire department's emergency number. A basic life-support truck and an advanced life-support rescue squad arrived at the scene at about the same time. Only twelve minutes had elapsed since the initial call was placed.

The paramedics noted that he was in distress, suffering squeezing substernal chest pressure, a feeling of "light-headedness," and slight shortness of breath. They immediately placed a nonrebreathing face mask giving him almost 100% oxygen. He was attached to a cardiac monitor and an intravenous line was started with 5% dextrose in water at a keep-open rate. By that time, his pain had subsided slightly and his vital signs included blood pressure 110/50, pulse 56, and respirations 22. His skin had dried and become warm. His lungs had some bibasilar rales. He reported that he had a history of hypertension and was taking some medication for it. He smoked and had a family history of heart attacks.

The paramedics then called the emergency department physician on duty for further orders (on-line medical control). They were told to administer one nitroglycerin tablet sublingually and repeat the vital signs. This produced further relief of his pain, but his pressure dropped to 96/50, and he became more light-headed. They were then told to give a fluid challenge of 300 ml of normal saline and to place the patient in a shock position. His pressure came up to 124/64 and he felt better. He was transported to the hospital in the supine position and had no further pain until he was about to be unloaded from the ambulance.

At this time his pulse was noted to be 40, his skin was cool and clammy again, and his chest pain recurred. The ED physician was called out to the ambulance ramp to see the patient, and immediately ordered a bolus of atropine given by intravenous push. This was done on the ambulance ramp while the patient was being wheeled into the department. While being pushed from the entrance of the department to the cardiac booth, his cardiac rate increased to 100, and some premature ventricular contractions appeared. An intravenous bolus of lidocaine was given, and he was transferred to the stretcher.

When he was transferred to the stretcher, he complained of increasing chest pain again, and within minutes his rate had slowed again to 44 with a sinus rhythm. He was given another dose of atropine and his rate again increased to 110. His blood pressure was then 120/62. He was given another nitroglycerin tablet, and morphine sulfate was ordered in case his pain continued. A twelve-lead ECG was begun, but before it could be completed, the patient slumped unconscious and was seen to be in ventricular fibrillation.

Two precordial chest thumps were administered while the defibrillator was charged, and the patient was ventilated with a bag-valve-mask on 100% oxygen. An initial shock was delivered at 200 joules, but the rhythm showed no change. A second shock delivered at 300 joules and a third at 360 joules produced no change in the rhythm. Cardiopulmonary resuscitation (CPR) was begun after the first shock and his trachea was intubated after the third shock. Epinephrine was given intravenously and he was shocked again at 360 joules with no change in his rhythm. After each shock it was observed that the fibrillatory waves were of lower amplitude. Lidocaine was given by intravenous bolus and he was shocked again. His rhythm deteriorated to asystole.

He was given another dose of epinephrine and atropine, and CPR and ventilations were continued. Since there was no change and he was young, the staff doctor elected to attempt transthoracic cardiac pacing. While this was being set up, another dose of epinephrine was given. The pacer functioned but the patient's heart did not capture the paced beats. Further attempts at treatment with intravenous epinephrine and atropine were unsuccessful, and he was pronounced dead about seventy-five minutes after arriving at the hospital.

Do the paramedics waste time by treating patients "in the streets"?

What are the priorities in a cardiac arrest? (hint: ABC)

DISCUSSION   Most patients who suffer cardiac arrest are found to be in ventricular fibrillation when a rhythm can be determined. The
chance of successfully defibrillating such a patient falls off rapidly with time. Early defibrillation is essential. There is indeed a
hazard in shocking a patient who has no palpable pulse due to
hypotension or supraventricular arrhythmias: The same ventricular fibrillation thought to be present initially may be
brought about by the shock. In some EMS systems, the standing
protocol is to shock the pulseless patient first and look at the
rhythm later. New, automatic external defibrillators will automatically determine the rhythm and shock only ventricular fibrillation.

An ambulance crew properly planned to handle emergency
resuscitation would consist of at least three persons. Most cities
use existing services, usually fire departments, to provide basic
and advanced life-support services. Many cities have initiated
citizen CPR programs that train a large portion of the population to perform one- and two-person CPR. Often, however, the
first responder in these cases is the basic EMT on a fire truck.
The second responder is the paramedic or advanced EMT on a
specially equipped rescue vehicle. Paramedics are trained to
recognize and initiate treatment of many life-threatening cardiac
problems. Most paramedics have between 700 and 1500 hours
of training including arrhythmia interpretation and observation
in the coronary care units. Treatment is often begun on the
scene by paramedics, and they will frequently delay transport of
a cardiac patient until the initial treatment is begun. Transport
can be done by these units or by a simultaneously dispatched
ambulance. The crew needs skills in ventilation with Ambu bag
and oral airway. They need good cardiac massage technique
and a van-type vehicle large enough to work over the patient
on the trip. They need intravenous infusion capabilities including sufficient height inside the vehicles to provide a pressure
head for intravenous infusions. Drugs usually carried are
$NaHCO_3$, atropine, lidocaine, epinephrine, bretylium, dop-
amine, isoproterenol, Lasix, morphine, naloxone (Narcan), glucose, glucagon, calcium, bicarbonate, and verapamil. The present standard of prehospital care is very high, and in some cities
over 40% of victims of ventricular fibrillation can now survive
to hospital discharge because of the rapid care delivered by
paramedics. The prognosis for patients presenting in asystole or
electromechanical dissociation remains dismal.

Once in the ED, a pulseless patient is resuscitated in a standardized fashion. Most important, one physician must take

charge of the procedure. Seldom should any voice but his be heard, and he should not be involved directly in carrying out the procedures, but should observe and command the entire team.

Advanced Cardiac Life Support (ACLS) teaches the principles of cardiac resuscitation through intensive courses. The Megacode is a lifelike simulation of a cardiac arrest performed on a mannequin with simulated arrhythmias. This training allows all persons involved in the care of patients in cardiac arrest to function smoothly as a team and eliminates much of the confusion that accompanied cardiac arrests in the past.

The following steps outline the American Heart Association's ACLS approach to cardiac arrest:

A. Attempt to reestablish spontaneous cardiac activity.
   1. In monitored ventricular fibrillation, a blow to the chest (precordial thump) may restore spontaneous activity.
   2. Follow this with three successive shocks of 200, 300, and 360 joules if earlier treatment is not successful.
B. CPR (one physician assumes the role of resuscitation chief).
   1. Suction airway when needed, place oral airway, and ventilate with 100% oxygen using a mask and Ambu bag to preoxygenate before intubation.
   2. Cardiac compressions start at about 100 per minute while a second person ventilates at about 20 per minute. Basic CPR must continue throughout the resuscitation efforts, pausing only momentarily to allow electric shock delivery and rhythm determination.
   3. Intubate the trachea with an endotracheal tube.
   4. Evaluate effectiveness of ventilation and massage.
C. Establish access and data base.
   1. IV, large bore if possible.
   2. ECG monitor with defibrillator capabilities.
   3. Blood gas on a stat basis.
D. Team leader evaluates the data obtained and the effectiveness of therapy.
E. Attempt definitive therapy. Continue massage and ventilation.
   1. Ventricular fibrillation.
      a. Epinephrine 1 mg (1:10,000) IV.
      b. Defibrillate at 360 joules.
      c. Lidocaine 1 mg per kg IV.
      d. Defibrillate at 360 joules.
      e. Bretylium 5 mg per kg IV.

     f. Defibrillate at 360 joules.

     g. Repeat lidocaine or bretylium.

     h. Give bicarbonate only based on the results of arterial blood gas measurements.

     i. Lidocaine or bretylium infusions should be started after the establishment of a supraventricular rhythm.

2. Asystole.

     a. Epinephrine 1 mg (1:10,000) IV every five minutes.

     b. Atropine 1 mg IV (repeated in five minutes).

     c. Consider external (transthoracic) pacemaker.

3. Electromechanical dissociation (EMD) (electrical rhythm but no pulse).

     a. Epinephrine 1 mg (1:10,000) IV every five minutes.

     b. Look and treat for treatable causes of EMD, such as pericardial tamponade, tension pneumothorax, severe hypovolemia, acidosis, hypoxemia, or pulmonary embolism.

4. Bradycardia or AV block.

    If hypotensive, accompanied by chest pain, or with ventricular escape beats, treat the patient, otherwise observe.

     a. Atropine 0.5–1.0 mg IV.

     b. External pacemaker or isoproteronol IV infusion.

     c. In an otherwise stable patient with third-degree or second-degree type II heart block, a transvenus pacemaker is the treatment of choice. The external pacemaker should be on standby while it is being arranged.

Unfortunately, as in this case, sometimes the best we can offer is still too late or too little. After a failed resuscitation effort involving a large team of people, we all may feel depressed. Then there is still a difficult task at hand. This man's family needs to be told the bad news; another painful challenge for the emergentologist.

REFERENCES

Textbook   Tintinalli. Pp. 3–104.

Review Article   Standards and guidelines for cardiopulmonary resuscitation and emergency cardiac care. *J.A.M.A.* 1986;255:2915–2984.

Additional References   Norto, J. P. New standards and guidelines for CPR and emergency cardiac care. *Am. J. Emerg. Med.* 1986;4:192–193.

Schmidt, T. A., and Tolle, S. W. Emergency physicians' responses to families following patient death. *Ann. Emerg. Med.* 1990;19:125–128.

Weaver, W. D. et al. Considerations for improving survival from out-of-hospital cardiac arrest. *Ann. Emerg. Med.* 1986;15:1181–1186.

Young, G. P. Reservation and recommendations regarding sodium bicarbonate administration in cardiac arrest. *J. Emerg. Med.* 1988;6:321–323.

Case 91 Thirty-Six Years Old, Fainted at the Office

A 36-year-old man fainted at his office and was brought to the emergency department by ambulance. When he arrived, he claimed to feel well and to be ready to return to work. He said that a bout of nervousness at work had apparently led him to pass out and that he had no other symptoms; however, a friend who had accompanied him to the hospital pointed out that at lunch one hour earlier the patient had complained of a severe pain in his upper midabdomen. The patient did then admit to a little stomach upset but no pain. He had never before suffered from pains of any sort, including heartburn, gas pains, or indigestion. He had never before had a similar spell of nervousness or faintness. He was on no drugs and was otherwise well. He drank only occasionally and did not smoke.

On physical examination, the patient was observed to be perspiring heavily. Blood pressure was 100/80 supine and 90/70 seated. The patient pointed out that his blood pressure was always low, although he did not know the usual numbers. His pulse was 110 supine and unchanged when he sat up. There were no other remarkable findings. An intravenous infusion was started, and nasal oxygen was administered. An ECG was taken and read as normal. The physician caring for this patient thought that he probably had had a myocardial infarction and admitted him to the coronary care unit. No rectal exam had been done because of the admitting diagnosis in the ED.

What are the usual reasons for profuse diaphoresis?

What danger is there in doing a rectal exam when the patient has had a myocardial infarction?

What is the diagnosis in this case?

DISCUSSION   Diaphoresis usually means hypoglycemia, shock, extreme ex-
penditure of energy such as in a laboring asthmatic, or a very
hot environment. It is also frequently seen in patients with acute
myocardial infarctions, acute pulmonary edema, or severe abdominal or back pain such as renal or biliary colic. True diaphoresis is a significant clinical finding and should always be
considered a sign of significant organic disease.

This patient was in a cool room and was neither dyspneic nor
laboring to breathe. A blood sugar was drawn, and 50 ml of
50% glucose solution was given intravenously. His condition
did not change, and the blood sugar was later reported to be
normal. This patient had hypotension of unknown cause. There
was no history of causative medications (antihypertensives,
beta blockers, diuretics, or narcotics); no history of dehydration
or bleeding to suggest hypovolemia; no spinal injury causing
neurogenic peripheral loss of tone; and no chest pain, ECG
changes, or heart failure to suggest cardiogenic shock. In this
setting of hypotension without an obvious cause, one needs to
consider occult septicemia (e.g, early urosepsis from an unsuspected urinary tract infection) and occult blood loss.

It has been shown that a gentle rectal exam imposes very
little stress in the presence of a fresh myocardial infarction, and
such an exam should be done. In this case the cause of the
fainting, sweating, and borderline hypotension was not clear,
and occult bleeding must be considered. Indeed, the patient
passed a large black diarrheal stool two hours later, and the
problem was clarified. His bleeding duodenal ulcer was easily
managed, and he did well subsequently. No further evidence of
a myocardial infarction ever appeared.

Peptic ulcer disease commonly presents with pain in the midepigastrium. If more blood is found on a rectal exam than just a
trace positive guaiac test, the patient should have a nasogastric
tube passed to help determine the site and extent of bleeding. If
there is bright red blood from the stomach, the bleeding is
active, and measures such as continued irrigation and administration of intravenous H_2-blockers such as cimetidine should be
begun. (If coffee-ground material is returned, the bleeding is
old; if it quickly clears and the patient's hematocrit is normal, he
may be a candidate for discharge and outpatient therapy.)

Lower gastrointestinal bleeding, although usually slow, can
be life-threatening in some situations. Patients should be checked for orthostatic changes in their vital signs and should have a
spun hematocrit determination. If the bleeding is by history
alone, and these two screening tests are normal, the patient

may be discharged and worked up as an outpatient.

Patients frequently deny serious significance to their symptoms. Denial is understandable but should not mislead the physician. Indeed, the admitting physician in this case was sure that he was dealing with serious cardiovascular illness even though the exact diagnosis was uncertain.

REFERENCES

Textbook   Rosen. Pp. 1418–1432.

Review Article   Schaffner, J. Acute gastrointestinal bleeding. *Med. Clin. North Am.* 1986;70:1055–1066.

Additional   Hickey, M. S., Kiernan, G. J., and Weaver, K. E. Evaluation of
Reference   abdominal pain. *Emerg. Med. Clin. North Am.* 1989;7:437–451.

Case 92 Recent Bypass Surgery

A 59-year-old man was discharged home from the hospital after having a coronary artery bypass graft done several days earlier. Two hours after discharge, he arrived in the emergency department complaining of substernal chest pressure and a pounding in his chest. He denied shortness of breath. His only medication was Tylenol with codeine for incisional pain.

On examination he appeared to be in no distress, but his face was pasty in color. He stated that the pain stopped when oxygen was applied via a nonrebreathing face mask. Vital signs were blood pressure 124/80, pulse 188, respirations 18, and temperature 98.6°F. The remainder of the physical examination was normal.

The patient was placed on a cardiac monitor, and the rhythm was interpreted as a narrow complex tachycardia with what appeared to be P waves preceding each beat. On this basis, he was given a 5-mg dose of intravenous verapamil. This had no effect on the rate. Carotid sinus massage likewise had no effect on the rate. A twelve-lead ECG was done at this time and showed a wide complex tachycardia. The patient was then given 100 mg of intravenous lidocaine. Several minutes later his heart rate slowed to 100 per minute. He was placed on a lidocaine drip and transferred to the coronary care unit.

How can you differentiate supraventricular from ventricular tachycardia?

What are the complications of supraventricular tachycardia and its treatment?

DISCUSSION   This patient presented with symptoms attributable to a tachyarrhythmia. This symptom complex may range from vague feel-
ings of apprehensiveness and fear to mental status changes,
seizure from lack of blood supply, and full cardiac arrest.

Patients with tachyarrhythmias who present to the ED and
are hemodynamically unstable should undergo immediate synchronized cardioversion, usually starting at 50 to 100 joules of
energy. The usual indications include hypotension (systolic
blood pressure less than 80), unconsciousness or obtundation,
pulmonary edema, or other signs associated with a poor cardiac
output. Chest pain alone may be enough to prompt electrical
cardioversion from a tachyarrhythmia. Synchronized cardioversion is the safest and most reliable way to terminate tachyarrhythmias in these patients.

In a more stable patient, the physician should proceed to
define the arrhythmia by careful assessment of the ECG and
physical exam. Most patients tolerate supraventricular tachycardias better than ventricular tachycardias. Usually our diagnostic
problem involves a wide QRS tachycardia (initially missed in
this case), and our challenge is to differentiate a supraventricular arrhythmia with aberrant ventricular conduction from ventricular tachycardia. (Aberrancy occurs when a supraventricular
reentrant impulse arrives at the AV node while one or both
bundle branches are refractory, and results in a widened QRS
complex.) The treatment of these two entities in the hemodynamically stable patient is quite different. Misdiagnosis and
subsequent inappropriate treatment have resulted in patient
deaths.

ECG evidence favoring a diagnosis of ventricular tachycardia
includes the presence of atrioventricular disassociation, a QRS
complex greater than 0.14 seconds, the appearance of fusion or
capture beats, concordance (all QRS complexes upright or all
inverted in the precordial leads), a marked left-axis deviation,
and the presence of RSr' in lead V_1. Findings on physical exam
suggesting the diagnosis of ventricular tachycardia include the
presence of cannon a-waves in the neck, varying loudness of
the first heard sound, and beat to beat variability in the systolic
blood pressure. Advanced age and a history of underlying coronary artery disease favor a diagnosis of ventricular tachycardia.

Once the diagnosis of ventricular tachycardia has been made,
appropriate initial management would include administration of
intravenous lidocaine or procainamide.

In those cases where the diagnosis of supraventricular tachycardia (SVT) is likely, vagal maneuvers may be useful. Car-

otid sinus massage, Valsalva maneuver, and the diving reflex (immersion of the patient's face into ice-cold water) are procedures that increase vagal tone and thereby prolong refractoriness at the AV node. This may aid in differentiating the type of SVT (atrial fibrillation versus atrial flutter versus paroxysmal SVT) and in some cases will abruptly terminate the arrhythmia. Carotid massage may be hazardous in an elderly or atherosclerotic patient. If vagal maneuvers are unsuccessful, verapamil administered by slow intravenous injection at a dosage of 0.075 mg per kg has been shown to be effective in terminating supraventricular tachycardias. Verapamil should be used cautiously in patients with a history of congestive heart failure, hypotension, or heart block. It has been shown to accelerate conduction over accessory pathways in patients with the Wolff-Parkinson-White (WPW) syndrome accompanied by atrial fibrillation.

Procainamide has also been shown to be effective in terminating both ventricular tachycardias and atrial tachycardias with aberrancy. In those cases of wide-complex tachycardia where the diagnosis remains unclear, it is best to choose between intravenous procainamide (if the patient is stable) or cardioversion (if the patient is not). That is because the diagnosis could be WPW syndrome with uncontrolled rapid atrial fibrillation and aberrancy; and lidocaine, digitalis, and verapamil can all lead to more rapid conduction through the accessory pathway and death in this setting.

REFERENCES

Textbook Schwartz. Pp. 907–930.

Review Article Benditt, D. G., et al. Supraventricular tachycardias: Mechanisms and therapies. *Hosp. Pract.* August 15, 1988;161–185.

Additional References Lowenstein, F. R., and Harken, A. H. A wide, complex look at cardiac dysrhythmias. *J. Emerg. Med.* 1987;5:519–531.

Moore, G. P., and Munter, D. W. Wolff-Parkinson-White syndrome: Illustrative case and brief review. *J. Emerg. Med.* 1989;7:47–54.

Case 93 Patient Who Became Loud and Abusive

A 34-year-old man presented himself to the triage nurse complaining of severe low back pain. He was moaning and groaning and appeared in such severe distress from his pain that the nurse immediately triaged him to a booth. He was promptly seen by a nurse and a senior emergency medicine resident.

He stated that the pain began a few days earlier and was the result of an exacerbation of an old injury. It started while he was lifting heavy packages at work. He had had numerous operations for slipped discs in the past. He had no neurologic deficit but told the staff that the pain felt exactly like his last slipped disc. He begged for some pain medication. He was taking no medication at the time but had used Percodan in the past. He said that he was allergic to codeine and requested a prescription for more Percodan.

Examination was difficult because of the patient's writhing and groaning, but the resident noticed that the patient could be distracted and showed no sign of pain when he sat up with his legs extended before him, a form of "straight leg raising." The physician suspected that his patient was seeking narcotics and told him that there was no indication of a disc herniation and narcotics were not needed. The patient was instead given a muscle relaxant and ibuprofen at which point he became angry and demanded "proper treatment" from the resident. The patient threatened to sue the resident, the nurse, and the hospital if he was not given the medication of his choice.

Distressed by the deteriorating situation, the resident asked for assistance from the attending physician on duty. This physician was equally unable to define the patient's level of pain and reproduced the resident's inconsistent findings on examination. The patient was again told that the use of narcotics in his case was inappropriate and that the resident's prescriptions should help for muscle spasms of the lower back. The patient, now loudly abusive of the physicians, shouted that he was going to sue the hospital and that the care given in the emergency department was substandard. The patient was told that if he was unsatisfied with the care, he was free to go to another hospital and get a second opinion. He then got dressed and left the department.

Later, the triage nurse reported to the physicians that as soon as the patient was outside the department and thought that he could no longer be seen by anyone inside, he began walking normally and appeared to be in no distress. The attending physician notified the neighboring EDs to be on the alert for this man should he show up in their departments seeking narcotics.

What is the function of the triage nurse?

How do drug seekers usually present?

What is the likelihood that he will sue?

DISCUSSION   By their nature, EDs must be available to everyone who seeks
care, twenty-four hours a day, and without regard to the patient's ability to pay. This makes them targets for persons seeking drugs for nonmedical or recreational purposes. Drug seekers often simulate low back pain, headache, or renal colic, and
it is difficult to separate those patients who are seeking drugs
from those with legitimate pain. Some subtle clues to drug-
seeking behavior include the lack of or contradictory objective
findings, "allergies" to non-narcotic analgesics or to codeine,
and "allergy" to contrast medium, which makes an intravenous
pyelogram impossible. These patients often demand immediate
relief of their pain, and they usually have no physician available
with whom telephone consultation can be made. Patients feign-
ing renal colic have been known to bite their tongues and spit
the blood into their urine specimen to mimic hematuria.

Some patients will threaten to sue if their demands are not
met. This is almost always an idle threat. If the diagnosis and
treatment are appropriate, the patient has no grounds to sue for
malpractice. Patients who appear to be in pain but have puz-
zling aspects to their story can be given a two-day supply of
medication and instructed to seek followup care within those
two days. If no narcotic medication is prescribed, the provider
should explain that the desired medication is too strong for this
problem and is not medically indicated, but that another analgesic can be used. There is very little to be gained by confronting
the patient in most ED encounters. In many cases the EDs will
warn each other and the patient's physician when they suspect
drug-seeking behavior. When they realize that access to these
drugs has been limited, these patients have been known to
move on to other cities.

When a patient walks into our ED, he first gives his complaint
to a triage nurse. The nurse has guidelines with which to sort
patients to different areas of the department. Inside our department a nursing assessment is performed and documented on
every patient. The nurse often uncovers facts that the patient is
hesitant to tell the doctor. A physician who fails to read the nursing notes on a patient does so at his own and his patient's peril.

REFERENCES
Textbook   Schwartz. Pp. 671–680.

Review Article   Dubin, W. R. Evaluating and managing the violent patient. *Ann.
Emerg. Med.* 1981;10:481–484.

Additional   Johnson, R., and Trimble, E. C. The (expletive deleted) shouter.
References   *JACEP* 1975;4:333–335.

Grove, J. E. Taking care of the hateful patient. *N. Engl. J. Med.*
1978;298:883–887.

Schwenk, P. L., et al. Physician and patient determinants of
difficult physician patient relationship. *J. Fam. Pract.* 1989;
28:59–63.

Case **94** Multiple Shooting Victims

The EMS dispatcher called in on the ambulance radio that there was a multiple-casualty incident in progress. Multiple shootings had occurred in a poor section of the city. Her initial report stated that there were at least five casualties. She heard that one might be dead at the scene; one had head, chest, and abdominal wounds; and there were several others. The trauma teams and several additional residents were called to the department to help in the anticipated disaster.

The department staff contacted the local police dispatcher to get more detailed information but none was available at the time. About twenty minutes later, a city paramedic unit called in on the medical control radio with the condition of one of the victims. They reported a man in his twenties who had been shot once in the head and was now unconscious. They had intubated his trachea, placed a large-bore intravenous line of Ringer's lactate, and were transporting him to the emergency department with an estimated time of arrival of five minutes. Indeed, in five minutes the team arrived with their announced patient, who had suffered a single gunshot wound to the head. They reported that there were other victims, but they had no idea of how many or the extent of their injuries.

Moments later, a second paramedic unit brought in another man in his twenties who had been shot once in the neck. He seemed to be breathing adequately. He had been treated in the field with two large-bore intravenous lines of lactated Ringer's and placed on oxygen with a nonrebreather mask.

The second paramedic unit reported that one person was declared dead on the scene, but they did not know if there were any other victims. Further radio calls to the dispatcher were made, but she had no further information about the incident.

When the police supervisor at the scene arrived about fifteen minutes later, he informed the ED team that these were the only living victims of the shooting. Another victim was pronounced dead at the scene, and they were still searching for other victims. They also knew of another incident, unrelated to this one, in which a man jumped out of a second-story window to avoid being shot. He was being transported to our department and arrived shortly thereafter.

The first patient, with the head injury, was rushed off to a CT scan, which showed widespread intracranial damage. He was placed on a ventilator, hyperventilated, and admitted but was declared brain dead several hours later. He was hepatitis B positive and thus unsuitable for organ donation. The second victim's wounds were explored in the ED under local anesthesia and the bullet track found to pierce the platysma muscle. He was admitted to the operating room for a neck exploration.

What is a multiple-casualty incident?

What are the elements of a disaster plan?

What are the priorities in treating penetrating injuries of the neck?

DISCUSSION   An *EMS disaster* is defined as a sudden calamitous event, producing injury and death that are beyond the capacity of the
normal EMS response. It may be a natural event or it may be
human-made: building collapse, explosion, plane crash, fire, or
multiple victims of a major motor vehicle accident. In any case,
the events are sudden and result in many casualties. Most natural disasters disrupt communications in the area, making notification of hospitals difficult. Weather-related disasters usually
cause many moderate to minor injuries and a trickle of more
serious ones. Persons with serious injuries usually are not found
soon enough to be brought to medical attention. Human-made
disasters lead to a bolus of many serious injuries arriving rapidly since the area of the disaster is usually well defined and can
be quickly reached by police, fire, and medical rescue units.
Multicasualty incidents are "minidisasters" in that they can
stress the facilities of any one hospital if all the victims of the
incident are brought there.

The key to successful disaster management is proper command structure at the scene and coordinated communications.
The paramedics should recognize any multicasualty incident as
a disaster, and a senior member of the first squad on the scene
should be designated as the incident commander. This person
will designate the roles for each of the subsequent rescuers to
play in the rescue and transport and is in charge of all communications from the scene. One rescuer assumes the role of the
triage officer. This person goes from one victim to the next and
performs a primary assessment on each patient before determining the priority with which each will be managed. This person will also begin treatment of the ABCs for each patient in
need of an open airway and ventilation. Of course, such a
scenario assumes an adequate number of well-trained rescuers.
The triage officer should tag patients with color codes to direct
the next arriving rescue teams. Black tags are placed on anyone
who is without vital signs or considered unsalvageable. Red tags
are put on those with immediately life-threatening injuries and
designate the highest priority for treatment and transport; yellow and green tags are put on those with lesser injuries.

Immediately life-threatening (red) injuries usually involve the
respiratory and cardiovascular systems. Less serious injuries (yellow) include multiple fractures, and head trauma lacking signs of
increasing intracranial pressure. Green-tagged patients are the
"walking wounded" and can help themselves to get to the am-
bulances. Prompt notification of the hospital by the incident
commander is essential in allowing the hospital to ready itself

for the patients and to allocate resources to each patient. Notification should include the number of casualties in each category and the approximate time it will take to extricate and transport the first patient. The hospital should be updated frequently.

We encourage our prehospital providers to treat any multiple-casualty incident as a disaster so that they can practice the elements of the disaster plan. This includes any incident in which there are more than two victims. Through this kind of practice, they will be familiar with the practical aspects of the plan and will be able to execute it when a major disaster strikes. In addition many municipalities stage a major disaster drill once a year. This usually includes a hypothetical scenario with "patients" moulaged to appear as real injuries and then transported to the hospitals and "treated." The drill concludes with a critique by all the participants to find weaknesses in the plan and its operation.

The second patient in this "disaster" had a penetrating wound of the neck. These wounds are usually explored in the operating room if the tract of the bullet or knife penetrates the platysma muscle. Even apparently superficial neck wounds demand close observation because of the threat of expanding hematoma and undetected great vessel, tracheal, and esophageal injuries.

REFERENCES
Textbook   Tintinalli. Pp. 175–179.

Review Article   Mahoney, L. E., et al. Disaster medical assistance teams. *Ann. Emerg. Med.* 1987;16:354–358.

Additional References   Mahoney, L. E., and Rutershan, T. T. Catastrophic disaster and the design of disaster medical care systems. *Ann. Emerg. Med.* 1987;16:1085–1091.

Fain, R. M., and Schreirer, R. A. Disaster, stress and the doctor. *Med. Educ.* 1989;23:91–96.

Haynes, B. E., et al. A pre-hospital approach to multiple victim incidents. *Ann. Emerg. Med.* 1986;15:458–462.

Selden, B. S. Adolescent epidemic hysteria presenting as a mass casualty, toxic exposure incident. *Ann. Emerg. Med.* 1989;18:892–895.

Guss, D. A., et al. The impact of a regionalized trauma system on trauma care in San Diego County. *Ann. Emerg. Med.* 1989;18:1141–1145.

Case 95 Stabbing Victim with Hostile Entourage

A 22-year-old man walked into the emergency department loudly saying that he had been stabbed in the abdomen. He was accompanied by several very large friends. He was brought to the trauma room, but the physician and nurse there were unable to approach his bedside because his friends, who were now quite agitated, were protesting loudly that everyone should "stay cool" and keep away from their friend, whom they stated they were there to protect. In their words, "No one comes near him, OK?" When they were finally ushered out, the patient was noted to have a 1-inch long abdominal stab wound in the middle of his left upper quadrant.

What should be done next for the patient?

How do you distinguish a life-threatening stab wound from a worrisome but trivial cut?

DISCUSSION   This group ritual is fascinating and its significance is still unclear. Is there really a need for protection? Is a rival gang about to burst into your ED and cut or shoot up the patient and your staff? It has been known to happen. More frequently, the group bluster is a face-saving gesture and is best dealt with by gestures of respect but firm policy statements. We seldom lose by adopting a posture of respect and honor toward our patients and their family or friends.

Should someone present a case to you in emergency medicine and ask "What should you do first?," a good answer is always "ABCs" regardless of what the case is about. In this case, after the airway, breathing, and circulation were checked, the physician scanned the patient for any other signs of serious trouble: tachypnea, tachycardia, diaphoresis, cyanosis, ashen appearance, or distended neck veins. (Elevated jugular venous pressure is important in trauma since there are two syndromes that can kill the patient rapidly and show markedly elevated venous pressure: pericardial tamponade and tension pneumothorax.) In this case, ignorant as we are of the length of the knife or the direction it took, we need to consider the very real possibility that the heart, lung, or aorta may have been injured in addition to the intra-abdominal organs. The best emergency physicians always consider the worst possibilities. If you diagnose the patient's condition as being relatively benign each time a relatively benign-looking patient presents to you, you will almost always be right, except when you are very wrong.

Since this patient showed no signs of systemic or serious injuries, the physicians were left considering the problems of a young man with a stab wound that might have violated the peritoneal cavity. Trauma centers vary in the care of this kind of case. We anesthetize the area and do a "miniexploration." If the wound is clearly superficial, and we can see the bottom of the wound and are convinced that the peritoneal cavity has not been entered, we suture and discharge the patient. If we get deeper into the wound and are not sure how deep it goes, we abort the procedure and do a diagnostic peritoneal lavage. There are a number of techniques for peritoneal lavage, but all include infusing 1000 ml of Ringer's lactate or normal saline into the peritoneal cavity and then measuring the concentration of red blood cells (RBCs) in the fluid after it is drawn off. In penetrating trauma our primary question is "Has the peritoneum been entered?" Our cutoff for a positive tap in this setting is 10,000 RBCs per mm^3 in the lavage fluid. In our institution all patients with trauma that has penetrated into the abdomen are admitted for serial examination or explored. If the patient had been hemodynamically unstable, we bypass the wound exploration and lavage and send the patient directly to the operating room for a laparotomy.

For blunt abdominal trauma, the diagnostic peritoneal lavage plays a different role. If the patient has sustained major blunt abdominal trauma and is hemodynamically unstable, again the proper path is to the operating room. If the patient is awake and alert and repeatedly has no signs or symptoms of any abdominal injury, then the lavage is again unnecessary. The role of peritoneal lavage is in the equivocal patient—where there has been a significant history of trauma but we are unsure if there is serious injury. Examples include patients who are intoxicated, difficult to evaluate, comatose from head injury, or have unexplained hypovolemia or falling hematocrit; we often find the peritoneal lavage clarifying in such patients.

REFERENCES
Textbook   Rosen. Pp. 519–547.

Review Article   Henneman, P. L. Penetrating abdominal trauma. *Emerg. Med. Clin. North Am.* 1989;7:647–666.

Additional   Thompson, J. S., et al. The evolution of abdominal stab wound
References   management. *J. Trauma* 1980;20:478–484.

Moore, E. E., and Marx, J. A. Penetrating abdominal wounds. *J.A.M.A.* 1985;253:2705–2708.

Thal, E. R. Peritoneal lavage: Reliability of RBC count in patients with stab wounds to the chest. *Arch. Surg.* 1984;119:579–584.

Marx, J. A. Methods of diagnostic peritoneal lavage—Better to be safe. *Am. J. Emerg. Med.* 1989;7:452–453.

Case 96 The Exploding Car Battery

A 23-year-old man was charging his automobile battery improperly when it exploded in his face. His face was struck by the top of the battery and splashed with acid. On arrival at the emergency department, he complained of not being able to see. We took him to a large sink where we washed his face with cool water. He had redness and blistering on his cheeks, under both eyes, and on his eyelids. Swelling and ecchymosis were evident around his left eye.

Topical anesthetic drops were instilled in both eyes, and within half a minute he had less pain. Each eye was irrigated with 1 liter of normal saline. He was given 4 mg intravenous morphine for pain relief, and then his eyes were examined with a slit lamp. His right eye showed a superficial corneal abrasion over the center of the visual field. The left showed a small hyphema that could only be seen with the slit lamp. He was referred for ophthalmologic evaluation.

What problems can result in a sudden loss of vision?

Which types of eye trauma require specialty care by an ophthalmologist?

Is this patient likely to develop orbital cellulitis?

DISCUSSION   Sudden loss of vision is most commonly due to blunt or pene-
                   trating trauma. Less commonly it can be due to retinal artery
                   occlusion, temporal arteritis, retinal or vitreous hemorrhages,
                   retinal vein occlusion, optic neuritis, or retinal detachment. All
                   patients with visual complaints need to have a visual acuity
                   performed, and almost all of those with true sudden loss of
                   vision require a prompt ophthalmologic consultation for help
                   with diagnosis and/or treatment.

                   Almost all serious chemical burns to the eye are caused by
                   strong acids or alkalis. (Alkaline burns are more dangerous be-
                   cause the alkaline material seeps into the corneal epithelium,
                   and this results in both deeper injury and greater potential for
                   scarring.) In any chemical burn, the eye should be IMME-
                   DIATELY and copiously irrigated. Using a few drops of topical
                   anesthetic was essential in helping this patient keep his eye
                   open during irrigation. Either water or normal saline could have
                   been used. Following irrigation the pH of the conjugational sack
                   should be checked, and irrigation should be continued until it
                   returns to normal (pH 7.3 to 7.7). The eye should then be
                   examined using a slit lamp and a "blue light" with fluorescein
                   dye. If a thorough eye examination is normal except for con-
                   junctival irritation, we generally do not obtain ophthalmologic
                   consultation, although followup in twelve to twenty-four hours
                   is recommended.

                   Blunt trauma to the eye can cause acute vision loss due to
                   globe rupture, retinal detachment, and hyphema (blood in the
                   anterior chamber). If the trauma is deeper than the cornea,
                   immediate ophthalmologic consultation is required. If a tho-
                   rough examination shows that the injury is limited to a superfi-
                   cial corneal abrasion, treatment with an eye patch, a topical
                   antibiotic, and close followup usually suffice.

                   This patient certainly had the potential to develop an orbital
                   cellulitis (heralded by a warm, red, proptotic eye), but that
                   syndrome occurs mostly in children or the immunocomprom-
                   ised and usually is not preceded by obvious external trauma.
                   This patient would have been more likely to develop a superfi-
                   cial cellulitis of the lids and periorbital tissue. This man received
                   good followup care, followed his discharge instructions care-
                   fully, and recovered uneventfully.

REFERENCES
Textbook   Schwartz. Pp. 1153–1161, 1340–1345.

Review Article   Zun, L. S. Acute vision loss. *Emerg. Med. Clin. North Am.*
                      1988;6:57–72.

Additional   Joondeph, E. C. Blunt ocular trauma. *Emerg. Med. Clin. North*
References   *Am.* 1988;6:147–168.

                      Luebeck, D. Penetrating ocular injuries. *Emerg. Med. Clin. North Am.* 1988;6:127–146.

                      Luebeck, D., and Greene, J. S. Corneal injuries. *Emerg. Med. Clin. North Am.* 1988;6:73–98.

Case 97 Broke the Steering Wheel with His Chest

A 67-year-old man was in a motor vehicle accident. His car struck a tree at a high rate of speed, which broke the steering wheel and shattered the windshield. When the EMS unit arrived, he was combative, with a blood pressure of 100/60. They placed him in a MAST suit, started two large-bore intravenous lines, and applied a cervical collar. He was taken to the nearest hospital. In that emergency department, his blood pressure was 110/60 and he was given Valium because of his agitation. A chest x-ray showed seven rib fractures and he was promptly transferred to the local trauma center.

On arrival there he was still quite agitated and complained of chest pain. He had received oxygen via nasal cannula during transfer, and his initial arterial blood gas results at the trauma center were pH 7.14, pO_2 55, pCO_2 46. He was intubated and placed on a ventilator. Thirty minutes later his pO_2 had risen to 180 and his mental status had improved. A repeat chest x-ray showed a hemothorax on the right side and a slightly widened mediastinum. A chest tube was placed and 150 ml of blood returned. A peritoneal lavage was positive. A repeat chest x-ray done after the chest tube was inserted showed a further widening of the mediastinum to over 12 cm, with obliteration of the aortic knob and displacement of his nasogastric tube to the right. Because of those signs, the doctors caring for him thought he had a traumatic aortic tear. Signs of diaphragmatic rupture (hazy diaphragm shadow, air fluid levels in the chest) were absent. The patient was taken to the operating room where an aortic angiogram was performed. When the angiogram was normal, the surgeon proceeded with a laparotomy, during which the patient's ruptured spleen was removed. He was admitted to the intensive care unit for continued ventilation therapy.

What was the significance of this man's initial acidosis?

Why did he need to be intubated and mechanically ventilated?

DISCUSSION   Acidosis on an initial arterial blood gas frequently is the first noted sign of shock in a patient who is still able to maintain a relatively normal blood pressure. This patient's hypoxia was caused by his hemothorax and inadequate ventilation due to chest wall trauma. He had a flail chest: Multiple ribs were broken in two locations, rendering a section of his chest wall unstable. He needed to be intubated and mechanically ventilated because of his hypoxia and because positive pressure ventilation is the most effective way to keep a flail segment moving with the rest of the chest wall.

The most dramatic injuries from blunt chest trauma are rupture of the aorta or the heart. They produce immediate exsanguination. A laceration of the aorta still encapsulated by clot or the vessel adventitia, or both, typically presents with no symptoms and must be suspected when a widened mediastinum is seen on a chest x-ray. A partial tear of the aorta can result in delayed rupture, so it is important to promptly do an aortogram to rule in or out the diagnosis when it is suspected.

Myocardial contusion is another potentially fatal complication of blunt chest trauma. It is a poorly understood condition that can occasionally result in life-threatening arrhythmias. Major blunt chest trauma patients are always admitted to an intensive care setting, but we just do not know which "minor" chest injury patients need to be admitted for cardiac monitoring.

REFERENCES
Textbook   Tintinalli. Pp. 850–863.

Review Article   Wilson, R. E., et al. Non-penetrating thoracic injury. *Surg. Clin. North Am.* 1977;57.

Additional   Mattox, K. L. Thoracic trauma. *Surg. Clin. North Am.* 1989;69:
References   1–78.

Marconha, K. E., et al. Blunt chest trauma and suspected aortic rupture: Reliability of the chest radiographic findings. *Ann. Emerg. Med.* 1985;14:644–649.

Danne, P. D., et al. Emergency bay thoracotomy. *J. Trauma* 1984;24:796–802.

Kearney, P. A., Rouhana, S. W., and Burney, R. E. Blunt rupture of the diaphragm: Mechanism, diagnosis and treatment. *Ann. Emerg. Med.* 1989;18:1326–1330.

Healey, M. A., et al. Blunt cardiac injury: Is this diagnosis necessary? *J. Trauma* 1990;30:137–145.

Case 98 VD

A young man in his twenties walked into the emergency department and told the triage nurse that he was not feeling well and wanted to see the doctor. He was very vague about his complaints and finally said he thought he had something wrong with his kidneys. He was triaged to the nonacute area of the department. The nurse on duty took his vital signs (which were normal) and asked him a few questions about his illness. He refused to give her any information and said he would tell only the doctor about his problem.

When the physician came in, he admitted to burning on urination and a yellow-white discharge from his penis. He also admitted to recent intercourse with a woman who was not his usual sexual partner. The remainder of his history was unremarkable. Examination revealed some discharge at the penile meatus that was sent off for culture and a small amount smeared on a slide for gram staining. He had some shotty inguinal lymph nodes and his prostate and epididymis were normal. The gram stain demonstrated many white blood cells, some of which were loaded with gram-negative intracellular diplococci.

He was treated with one dose of 250 mg ceftriaxone intramuscularly and 100 mg of oral doxycycline bid for ten days. Blood was drawn for syphilis serology, and he was instructed to go to the state venereal disease (VD) clinic six weeks later for repeat serology and culture. He was also told to have his recent sexual contacts examined and treated for gonorrhea and *Chlamydia* infections, and to avoid sexual intercourse for a week to ten days.

What diagnostic techniques are used to detect sexually transmitted diseases?

If this patient's sexual partners are not clearly identified and diagnosed, will they be sure to seek therapy because of their own symptoms? If not, what will happen to them?

Could this have been syphilis? Herpes?

DISCUSSION   In most men with either gonorrhea or *Chlamydia,* there is symptomatic evidence of VD, although the patient may be reluctant to describe the symptoms even to the physician. In contrast, most women with gonococcal or chlamydial cervicitis show no symptoms, perhaps for months or years. Nonetheless, if therapy is withheld, the patient may well go on to develop acute pelvic inflammatory disease (PID) or distant septic spread such as gonococcal arthritis.

The patient should be examined. In men the urethra should be cultured by taking a specimen from the vault just inside the meatus. In women, the cervical os should be cultured (after an initial swabbing to remove as much cervical mucus as possible). The next most useful sites for culture are the anal canal and the urethra, in that order. A gram stain of the cervix is not very helpful, for it is often negative when cultures are positive and sometimes falsely read as positive due to the presence of pleomorphic gram-negative rods which are normal flora *Neisseria vaginalis.*

Males presenting with penile discharge should have a gram stain made of their discharge. This may demonstrate the classic gram-negative intracellular diplococci and sheets of white blood cells typical of gonorrhea. If only white cells are present, the patient is presumed to have nongonococcal urethritis, usually caused by *Chlamydia.*

All men with symptoms suggestive of gonorrhea or *Chlamydia* need to be aggressively treated. Delaying treatment until culture results are available risks progression of the infection and nontreatment due to noncompliance. So, "Treat 'em while you got 'em." Treatment for both gonococcus and *Chlamydia* is recommended, as more than a fourth of patients with gonococcus also have *Chlamydia.* Because penicillin-resistant gonorrhea is becoming more frequent, the initial treatment of choice is now ceftriaxone 250 mg intramuscularly given once, followed by doxycycline 100 mg orally bid for seven days. Since the incidence of syphilis is rising, and it is not adequately treated with this regimen, a VDRL or equivalent serologic test for syphilis should be obtained at the time of treatment.

The most common complication of untreated or inadequately treated gonorrhea in either sex will be a persistent subclinical infection with the patient still able to transmit the disease. Female carriers may at any time become acutely ill with PID and develop nausea, vomiting, lower abdominal pain, tenderness, fever, leukocytosis, or rebound tenderness with peritonitis, all of which make differentiation from appendicitis difficult. This acute pelvic inflammatory disease may require hospitalization with parenteral high-dose antibiotic therapy and may render her sterile thereafter. It will also predispose her to future ectopic pregnancies. Such an acute illness may develop weeks or months after the initial contact with gonorrhea, thus treatment of asymptomatic gonorrhea is essential. In fact, therapy without a pelvic examination would be acceptable even if not optimal. We automatically treat known sexual contacts of patients who have gonorrhea. We do not wait for the results of the culture to begin therapy when there is a suggestive history as in this case.

Occasionally syphilis or herpes genitalis can be diagnosed in the ED, and the incidence of both infections has increased dramatically over the past few years. Syphilis can be detected in the early stage by the presence of a painless ulcer (chancre) in the genital area. Confirmation by dark-field microscopy can be difficult for most labs, and presumptive treatment with benzathine penicillin is often undertaken. A more common cause of venereal ulceration is herpes genitalis. It usually presents with a small cluster of vesicles or ulcers that are extremely painful. The diagnosis can be confirmed by a Tzank smear (which is much like a PAP smear) or by culture. Early treatment with acyclovir topically or systemically, or both, can shorten the duration of the symptoms in some cases, especially first episodes. In patients like this man, with a discharge but no ulcerations, we do not pursue diagnostic testing for herpes, but we do routinely check a VDRL syphilis serology.

REFERENCES
Textbook   Tintinalli. Pp. 674–676.

Review Article   Horsburgh, C. R., Douglas, J. M., and Haraforce, F. M. Preventative strategies in sexually transmitted diseases for the primary care physician. *J.A.M.A.* 1987;258:815–821.

Additional   Treatment of sexually transmitted diseases. *Med. Lett.* 1988;30
References   (757):5–10.

McNabney, W. K., and Barnes, W. G. Urethral and endocervical cultures: Gonorrhea and chlamydia. *Ann. Emerg. Med.* 1986; 15:333–336.

Case 99 Cerebrovascular Accident

A 79-year-old man was brought to the emergency department of a community hospital by his worried wife. She said that he had awakened that morning and come down to breakfast but that his speech made no sense and he seemed as frustrated by the trouble as she was. He had been able to walk and could make words but they seemed "all wrong." As the day progressed, he had developed a clumsiness and had begun to drop things. Finally, after dinner, she had been so worried that she brought him into the hospital.

The patient had been well prior to that day. He was a retired air-conditioner repairman. He had not smoked, drank rarely, and was not noted to be allergic to any medicines. His usual physician, not yet called, had been treating the patient with digoxin and hydrochlorothiazide for "an irregular heart beat."

On examination, the patient was well nourished and appeared well except for the neurologic system. His blood pressure was 170/95, pulse 88 and largely regular, with a few irregularities that the emergency physician thought to be atrial premature beats. He was afebrile and his respiratory rate was 16. He was having a great deal of difficulty with his speech, making no sense at all. He could not name common objects (pen, comb, book) that were shown to him and seemed exasperated by his own difficulty. He managed to articulate "God damn it!" several times. His right arm and leg were both weak compared to his left side. There was a slight droop to the right side of his mouth, but when he tried to close his eyes very tightly, his mouth actually pulled up higher on the right side. He could follow simple commands but had difficulty with more complex requests such as "Touch your right ear with your left hand."

The ECG showed atrial fibrillation with a well-controlled ventricular rate.

The emergency physician called the patient's primary care doctor and they agreed that this patient was suffering a "stroke in evolution." The atrial fibrillation was a long-standing problem. The patient had also been noted to have mild hypertension in the past, well controlled with a small dose of a diuretic.

The primary care physician asked the ED doctor to admit her patient to the hospital. She would be in to visit in the morning. In the meantime, she asked, should the patient be anticoagulated?

What of anticoagulation for a "stroke in evolution"?

Where is this patient's lesion?

Should his blood pressure be lowered at this time?

DISCUSSION   This patient does seem to be suffering from a cerebrovascular accident, probably an infarction in the region of the left middle cerebral artery. In a patient with atrial fibrillation, the stroke may be of embolic origin, but may just as likely be thrombotic. He has right-sided hemiparesis and aphasia. The aphasia seems to be more expressive than receptive but has elements of both, as it usually does. It is still somewhat fluent as the patient can make words, even if they are inappropriate and make little sense. He is aware of his difficulty and distressed by it and will be appreciative of his doctor's recognition of that distress.

Differentiating aphasia from confusion can be difficult but important since aphasia is a local, usually left-sided phenomenon, and confusion usually denotes diffuse brain disease. The aphasic patient may be aware of his difficulty and may express his awareness and his distress quite emphatically and quite verbally. If he is not able to express it, he may still be receptive to your recognition and comments on his difficulty: Your saying, "You seem to be having a great deal of trouble with speech right now" may be met with vigorous nodding and a smile of relief. The aphasic patient may be able to pick the right word out of a list and then will have a tendency to use that word over and over, incorrectly, as new objects are shown to him or new questions posed. The aphasic patient will have more trouble following complex requests than simple ones, and requests that oblige him to cross the midline will be still more difficult.

Current dogma suggests that we should be gentle in treating hypertension after a stroke has occurred. The patient may have considerable brain swelling and may need a high pressure to perfuse his brain. In fact, plasma expanders are currently being used with some success to limit brain damage in such patients. We would not suggest decreasing this patient's blood pressure further during the acute phase of the cerebral infarction.

Anticoagulation therapy in such patients has been long debated and the data remain confusing. Of course, the patient in atrial fibrillaton has another reason for anticoagulation: not to effect this stroke, but to prevent another embolic event. The big question is whether treatment with anticoagulants prevents progression of a stroke in the midst of its usual evolution. The data are mixed and experts divided in their opinions. This patient was treated with heparin and then Coumadin, as well as oxygen. His initial CT scan was entirely normal. The hemiparesis developed further during his first three days in the hospital and the clinical diagnosis remained that of a left cerebral infarction. The radiologist commented that early CT scans are often normal in such strokes and that it would probably show an infarction if repeated in a week or two.

Ten days after the onset of the stroke, while in a rehabilitation program, with a prothrombin time of 18 seconds due to Coumadin therapy, the patient suddenly worsened. He became stuporous and developed Cheyne-Stokes respiration. A repeat CT scan of his brain at that time showed a large hemorrhagic infarction in his left frontoparietal cerebral cortex. There was a slight midline shift to the right. The lateral ventricles were distorted by mass effect. A consulting neurologist thought that an initial ischemic infarction had hemorrhaged, partly due to the anticoagulation, and recommended stopping the Coumadin and perhaps reversing its effect with fresh frozen plasma. The patient did not improve and was eventually discharged to a nursing home. Unfortunately, we have also seen a similar patient who was *not* anticoagulated then proceed to throw a second, more massive clot to his brain and do equally poorly. That is what makes the decision whether to anticoagulate or not so difficult.

REFERENCES
Textbook   Rosen. Pp. 1733–1749.

Review Article   Sherman, D. G., et al. Cerebral embolism. *Chest* 1986;89:(Suppl.):82s–98s.

Additional   Cutler, R. W. P. Cerebrovascular Diseases. In E. Rubenstein and
References   D. D. Fedderman (eds.), *Scientific American*. New York, Scientific American, 1986. Ch. II, X. Pp. 1–10.

Jonas, S. Anticoagulant therapy in cerebrovascular disease: Review and meta-analysis. *Stroke* 1988;19:1043–1048.

Case **100** Medical Malpractice

A 15-year-old student from a local boarding school was brought into the emergency department complaining of neck pain. She was accompanied by the school nurse who presented a signed consent from the youth's parents (both physicians) allowing treatment in case of emergency.

The student said that she had intermittent neck pains in the past and an exacerbation over the past two days without any trauma or other precipitating cause. Examination revealed no abnormalities except pain on palpation of the neck. In fact, the patient jumped when the paraspinous muscles were palpated. Treatment with acetaminophen, bedrest, and a cervical collar was recommended. She was discharged to the care of the school nurse.

Four years later the physician was presented with a charge of malpractice against this patient claiming that by his failure to take cervical spine x-rays and to perform proper treatment, the patient had continuous unremitting pain and was unable to pursue her chosen career as a surgeon.

What is the most appropriate ED workup and treatment for nontraumatic neck pain?

What are the elements of medical malpractice and who gets sued?

What are the best defenses against a successful malpractice suit?

DISCUSSION   Any physician can be sued for malpractice! The shock of being
sued in this case was that there was no real question about the
appropriateness of the treatment rendered. This suit was begun
four years after the incident (the statute of limitations began
again when the patient became 18). By that time the facts were
far from the memory of the practitioner. Malpractice accusa-
tions can come at any time and about any case. Sometimes a
patient who did not get the anticipated result or who had a poor
outcome wants to be paid for a perceived wrong. Sometimes
suits are brought by patients who do not get better or who get
worse and are angry about the outcome.

The elements of a successful medical malpractice suit are (1)
preexisting duty to treat, (2) breach of that duty, (3) damages
present, and (4) *"proximate cause."* Duty exists whenever any
person presents to the ED for treatment. Breach of duty includes any action that the physician performs or does not perform that is below a set standard of treatment for the problem.
The standard may be local or national. Damages are whatever
the patient alleges to have suffered. *Proximate cause* means
that the damage must have been caused by the breach of duty.
All four of these must be proven in court in order for a malpractice charge to be upheld. Where good samaritan acts apply
(e.g., when a physician stops by the side of the road to aid an
accident victim), different standards apply and malpractice is
harder to prove. In any case, the job of the lawyer arguing a
malpractice case is to convince a panel of ordinary citizens that
his or her client's damages are severe, will interfere with her life,
and that the physician may be at least partly to blame for the
damages.

Although this appears to paint a dismal picture of the physician's ability to defend against a malpractice case, many defen-
sive measures can be taken to prevent a bad outcome. *The
most important defense that the physician has is the medical
record.* A well-written and comprehensive description of the
events involved in the encounter will allow the physician to
reconstruct long-forgotten events and explain the reasons for
the treatment given. Equally important are the nursing notes
and prehospital care provider notes. These can all help corrob-
orate the physician's information. The importance of the medical record cannot be overemphasized, and it is reasonable to
treat every chart as if you were going to have to go to trial with
it in the future.

Poor outcomes in medical practice do occur, and these
should be documented along with the reasons for their occur-

rence. An active departmental quality assurance program will help to discover which types of cases have the greatest potential for malpractice action and allow the physicians to improve their treatment and documentation of these cases. In this case the physician and nurse had both documented the case carefully, and although the case went to trial, it was won by the physician. Had the documentation been poor, the outcome might have been different.

The workup for acute nontraumatic neck pain in an otherwise healthy young person depends on the setting. If increasing pain, neurologic signs, or hard, matted lymph nodes are present, an x-ray may be useful to look for underlying neoplastic disease of the spine. Otherwise, physical examination including range of motion, areas of tenderness, distal sensation, strength, and circulation are all that are necessary for a presumptive diagnosis. In older age groups, x-rays should be taken more freely because the incidence of bony metastases is higher, and the presence of osteoporosis increases the likelihood of cervical spine fracture with otherwise minimal trauma. Treatment is the same for acute muscle spasm or a herniated disc without cord or nerve root involvement. The treatment prescribed in this case was reasonable. We recommend followup in a week if needed. Further evaluation can then be performed as an outpatient.

REFERENCES

Textbook   Tintinalli. Pp. 644–649, 979–982.

Review Articles   Cailliet, R. *Neck and Arm Pain.* Philadelphia, Davis, 1964. Pp. 40–44, 86–90.

                        George, J. E. *Law in Emergency Care.* St. Louis, Mosby, 1980. Pp. 1–34, 96–120.

Additional   Gore, D. R., et al. Neck pain. A long term follow-up of 205
References   patients. *Spine* 1987;12:1–5.

                        Trautline, H., Lambert, R. L., and Miller, J. Malpractice in the emergency department: Review of 200 cases. *Ann. Emerg. Med.* 1984;13:709–711.

                        Medical Malpractice Statutes. Arizona Revised Statutes. St. Paul, MN, West, 1982. Pp. 357–370. (Describes a model malpractice statute.)

Appendix # Core Content for Undergraduate Education in Emergency Medicine*

KNOWLEDGE BASE

I. Orientation to emergency medicine
   A. Principles of emergency care
      1. Recognition of threats to life and limb: 4, 6, 8, 12, 19, 23, 25, 30, 32, 34, 42, 46, 47, 58, 59, 70, 71, 72, 74, 77, 78, 80, 85, 86, 87, 88, 91, 94, 95, 97
      2. Evaluation of the emergency department patient: 2, 5, 8, 9, 11, 19, 24, 30, 31, 34, 37, 40, 41, 42, 47, 48, 49, 52, 53, 55, 58, 62, 63, 65, 67, 69, 70, 74, 75, 76, 78, 79, 80, 85, 86, 87, 88, 91, 93, 95, 97, 100
   B. Emergency medical services
      1. Prehospital care: 1, 4, 13, 17, 35, 49, 53, 57, 61, 64, 68, 77, 83, 90, 97
      2. Model systems/local system: 4, 17, 35, 61, 64, 83, 90, 94
      3. Paramedic, EMT training and function: 1, 17, 35, 57, 61, 64, 68, 90, 94
      4. Regionalization/categorization of care/trauma centers/disaster planning/triage: 42, 68, 83, 94
II. Cardiovascular diseases
   A. Cardiopulmonary resuscitation
      1. One- and two-rescuer CPR: 13, 90
      2. Conscious and unconscious victim: 13, 87, 90
      3. Choking victim: 63, 87
      4. Infant CPR: 13, 14
   B. Advanced cardiac life support
      1. Coordination and priorities in cardiac arrest: 13, 14, 42, 86, 90

Appendix was adapted from Society of Teachers of Emergency Medicine, Core content for undergraduate education in emergency medicine. *Ann Emerg Med* 1985; 14(5):474–476.
*Numbers refer to cases.

335

F. Altered mental status: 4, 15, 19, 27, 31, 32, 35, 36, 37, 46, 47, 58, 70, 78, 99

XV. Musculoskeletal disorders

   A. Neurovascular extremity examination: 26, 50, 82

   B. Strains/sprains/fractures (recognition): 3, 38, 52, 55, 82, 93, 100

   C. Septic joint (recognition): 18, 38, 89

   D. Dislocations (recognition): 82

   E. Soft tissue injury/infection (recognition): 3, 38, 49, 50, 51, 52, 55, 60, 61, 82, 86, 89, 100

XVI. Behavioral emergencies

   A. Recognition of acute psychosis: 1, 33, 48, 58, 78

   B. Suicidal and homicidal evaluation: 1, 2, 41, 48, 77

   C. Recognition of behavioral disorders caused by organic illness: 4, 19, 21, 22, 24, 25, 27, 31, 33, 35, 37, 47, 58, 70, 78, 86

   D. Performance of mental status examination: 4, 19, 27, 33, 40, 41, 46, 58, 78

SKILLS

I. Laceration repair: 15, 50, 61

   A. Suture materials, needles, instruments: 15, 61

   B. Types of wounds: 15, 38, 61, 95

   C. Wound preparation: 15, 38, 50, 61

   D. Tetanus prophylaxis: 15, 38, 61

   E. Local anesthesia: 15, 61

II. Cardiopulmonary resuscitation: 13, 14, 42, 90

III. Megacode training (ACLS): 13, 14, 42, 72, 90

IV. Electric countershock

   A. Defibrillator operation: 42, 72, 90

   B. Indications: 42, 72, 90, 92

V. Vascular access: 14, 16, 23, 26, 68

VI. Airway control: 39, 87

   A. Bag-mask ventilation: 16, 73, 85, 90

   B. Intubation: 13, 14, 16, 17, 26, 48, 56, 67, 68, 73, 85, 90

   C. Cricothyroidotomy: 56, 63, 85

   D. Esophageal obturator airways: 13

VII. Splinting/immobilization: 3, 49, 82, 86

VIII. Cervical spine immobilization: 1, 49

IX. Gastric lavage: 13, 16, 34, 48, 77, 91

X. MAST suit application: 1, 57, 64, 68, 83, 97

XI. Superficial abscesses—incision/drainage: 51, 89

XII. Nasal packing: 23

**TOPICS NOT
OTHERWISE
LISTED**

Index